UNPAID CARE POLICIES IN THE UK
Rights, Resources and Relationships

Liz Lloyd

P

First published in Great Britain in 2025 by

Policy Press, an imprint of
Bristol University Press
University of Bristol
1-9 Old Park Hill
Bristol
BS2 8BB
UK
t: +44 (0)117 374 6645
e: bup-info@bristol.ac.uk

Details of international sales and distribution partners are available at
policy.bristoluniversitypress.co.uk

© Bristol University Press 2025

British Library Cataloguing in Publication Data
A catalogue record for this book is available from the British Library

ISBN 978-1-4473-6129-9 hardcover
ISBN 978-1-4473-6130-5 paperback
ISBN 978-1-4473-6131-2 ePub
ISBN 978-1-4473-6132-9 ePdf

The right of Liz Lloyd to be identified as author of this work has been asserted by her in accordance with the Copyright, Designs and Patents Act 1988.

All rights reserved: no part of this publication may be reproduced, stored in a retrieval system, or transmitted in any form or by any means, electronic, mechanical, photocopying, recording, or otherwise without the prior permission of Bristol University Press.

Every reasonable effort has been made to obtain permission to reproduce copyrighted material. If, however, anyone knows of an oversight, please contact the publisher.

The statements and opinions contained within this publication are solely those of the author and not of the University of Bristol or Bristol University Press. The University of Bristol and Bristol University Press disclaim responsibility for any injury to persons or property resulting from any material published in this publication.

Bristol University Press and Policy Press work to counter discrimination on grounds of gender, race, disability, age and sexuality.

Cover design: Nicky Borowiec
Front cover image: Adobe/jozefmicic

Contents

About the author   iv
Preface   v

1   Introduction and background to unpaid care in the UK   1
2   Research and knowledge development on unpaid care in the UK   15
3   Policies to support unpaid carers   36
4   Policies into practice   65
5   Analysis of policies in context   92
6   The political and ethical dimensions of care   114
7   Conclusions   134

References   146
Index   166

About the author

Liz Lloyd is Senior Research Fellow at the University of Bristol, having retired from her post as Professor of Social Gerontology in 2019. Her career has spanned teaching and research in gerontology, social work and social policy. Her research has focused on ageing, older people's experiences of care and social care policies. She is a fellow of the Academy of Social Sciences, a senior fellow of the National Institute for Health and Care Research School for Social Research and an associate editor of the *International Journal of Care and Caring*.

Preface

This book was planned shortly before the first COVID-19 lockdown in March 2020, a time of reappraisal in public perceptions of care. I had retired as Professor of Gerontology at the University of Bristol after almost 30 years of teaching and research, which coincided with the period covered in the book. During that time, unpaid care has featured in both my working and personal life and these reflections on policies are therefore also reflections on my career as an academic and on the development of my ideas about dependency and care. One of the most pleasurable aspects of writing the book has been reading and re-reading texts written by colleagues, co-researchers and co-authors and revisiting research projects that have stimulated different ways of looking at dependency and care. Equally pleasurable has been exploring the academic work of the remarkable individuals who I have advised or examined as postgraduate students, some of whom are cited in this text. I consider myself extremely fortunate to have had such opportunities, which have enriched my understanding of policies, practices and theories of care.

My thanks are due to many people who have been supportive during the writing of the book. First and foremost, I thank Wenjing Zhang for her generosity with her time and expertise in preparing the bibliography. I also thank Randall Smith, Ailsa Cameron, Paul Willis and other colleagues at the School for Policy Studies in the University of Bristol, who have been hugely stimulating and supportive colleagues over the past 24 years. I also thank the G8 group of gerontology researchers, who have helped sharpen my ideas about practice, and have given great advice.

Many thanks are due to Laura Vickers-Rendall, Jay Allan, Julia Mortimer and others at Policy Press for their unstinting support and guidance. They are a terrific team to work with.

My friends and family members have shared their own experiences of caring and have given me valuable insights into the meaning of supportive relationships. Thanks to you all.

Ed Cape has supported me throughout the process of writing and the book is dedicated to him.

1

Introduction and background to unpaid care in the UK

Introduction

On 4 March 2021, a day after the budget statement in the House of Commons, a discussion took place on the BBC's *World at One* programme. Carers, service users, politicians and professionals had reacted with disappointment and anger that despite unprecedented levels of pressure and financial hardship experienced by families and care workers throughout the COVID-19 pandemic there had been no mention of social care in the budget statement. Interviewed by Sarah Montague, Sir Andrew Dilnot, who had chaired the Commission on Funding of Care and Support in 2011 (Dilnot 2011), referred to the sorry state of social care in the UK as a 'stain on our nation'. He argued that funding for social care is affordable, despite the many calls on the nation's finances, but that 'courage and strength of will' were needed to develop a policy on social care. 'Why courage?' asked Sarah Montague. He replied, 'Because, for reasons that I don't fully understand, elderly people and working aged people and children needing this kind of care are not a subject we find it easy or comfortable to speak about'. And because social care is a subject that politicians would prefer to avoid, said Dilnot, 'we have allowed it to be in the margins, in the shadows of our society and our economic and social policy and that does us no credit'.

This exchange draws attention to the scope of debates on care policies, to the social, cultural and philosophical issues involved in caring. It provides valuable context for an analysis of policies on *unpaid* care. Indeed, it suggests that unpaid care is in a particularly perilous situation because with social care policies confined to the margins, unable to attract political attention or economic resources, pressures on unpaid carers will continue unabated. Policies are shaped by economic and political priorities and reflect dominant cultural values. Policies exist in decisions and actions as well as in the absence of these and the lack of attention to social care in the 2021 budget should be understood, therefore, as a purposeful policy decision, not an accidental oversight. In the autumn statement by the Chancellor of the Exchequer in November 2022, reform to social care was further postponed until 2025, causing Dilnot to query how social care could be placed at the bottom of the list of priorities in a statement that, it was claimed, prioritised the government's commitment to protecting vulnerable people (Dilnot 2022). Arguably, for a government primarily focused on curbing demands on public expenditure, social care is one of the easiest things to leave out because it is already in the margins. In their 2021 annual survey of unpaid carers, Carers UK referred to the intolerable pressures that they were experiencing, not only those arising because of the COVID-19 pandemic but also because of inadequate support from health and social care services over the longer term. Their report called for carers to be *recognised and valued for what they do* (Carers UK 2021a). That carers were calling for this in 2021, just as they were over 30 years previously, raises a series of questions, which stimulated the writing of this book. Why has this heavy load on unpaid care developed in a country that has a welfare system? Are carers engaged in a Sisyphean struggle to achieve their aims through government action? What has been the role and purpose of successive policies on unpaid care and what effect have they had on unpaid carers and those that need care and support?

The aim of this book is to reflect on and analyse trends in key policies on unpaid care, to examine these in the context of policies on social care but also at wider social and political levels. When care in the community was introduced, policies became an important focus of campaigns by unpaid carers, who sought government action for change in their circumstances. Their organisations have been active at the heart of policy making throughout that time and it is through this involvement that their voice has been influential in the design and direction of policies. There is, therefore, a two-way link between the growth of the carers' movement and policies on unpaid care, which increasingly came to be about how unpaid carers should be supported.

Unpaid care *relationships* are known to be widespread but knowledge about them is contentious and, as Dilnot observed, discussion of care needs provokes discomfort. It is also known that unpaid care is increasingly challenging, with longer hours and more complex activities demanded of those that provide it. Less often considered are the demands unpaid care places on those who require support and care, and the effects of these challenges on family relationships. Policies and practices have shaped perceptions and expectations of care and about the nature of dependency. Caring 'dyads' have emerged as the dominant picture in policies, in which one person cares for one other person, identified as dependent upon them. The carer might be offered training for the role and put in touch with others in similar circumstances, so solidifying their carer identity. In these circumstances, as Clare Beckett (2007) reminded us, care can be a disempowering experience for those that need it. As one person becomes a carer the other becomes a 'dependant', with associated loss of status. The role of policies in reinforcing these perspectives is a crucially important point.

Sevenhuijsen (1998) argued that policy texts can be understood as 'vehicles of normative paradigms'. Policy documents establish the public profiles of groups and enable their claims to be expressed in legitimate and acceptable ways. For unpaid carers in the UK, it would be fair to say that an enduring normative paradigm has been that of the carer as an 'unsung hero', not only because of their devotion to the individual they support but also because through their self-sacrifice they make a major contribution to society in general. The trouble with heroism, of course, is that the hero stands out from the crowd and the acts that made them heroic become their entire identity. It is not an easy or comfortable place to be, nor is it a place that carers have asked to be. Indeed, their campaigns have been about dispensing with the need for self-sacrifice through a higher income, better conditions of employment for those in work and improved support services. An alternative paradigm, typically seen in introductions to policies, is that unpaid care affects us all, that many of us will be carers and we never know when this will be. Carers are part of normal life as a widespread and diverse group in society. The corollary of this, of course, is that the need *for* care is widespread and affects us all in diverse ways. Recognition of the need for care as a universal human experience is also central to the analysis in this book.

A troubled history

The history of policies on unpaid care is peppered with conflicting perspectives and ambiguous statements. It is also characterised by repetition, the same statements and sentiments appearing again and again in documents and debates. These refer to carers' importance to the social care system; the increasing value of their contribution to society as the population ages; and the justice of their claim to be valued and supported. Also repeated throughout those 30 years are carers' experiences of being devalued, unrecognised, ignored, overlooked and taken for granted. In 1989, Jill Pitkeathley, then Director of the Carers National Association, argued that change depends on legislation, although she was aware of the evident contrast between the rhetoric and the reality of policies. She observed that 'it is not difficult to get policy makers, service providers, researchers, academics, government spokespersons and carers themselves to agree on what should be done for carers', but that getting done what should be done is another matter (Pitkeathley 1989: 150). She pointed to the Community Care Act, 1990 as an instance of this contrast. Government rhetoric acknowledged that care in the community depended on the contribution of unpaid carers, whose contribution merited support, but they then introduced changes that, as Pitkeathley observed, would 'further impoverish and disadvantage carers' (Pitkeathley 1989: 167). In response to the question of why there is this gap, she considered a range of 'insoluble conflicts' beyond the sphere of policy making, which impede recognition of carers. These included the sense of obligation felt by carers to keep their relatives out of institutional care and the potential for conflicts of interest within care relationships; conflicts with professionals who lack respect for and recognition of carers; the societal need for carers and the likely reduction in the availability of carers; and the stereotyping of women as carers. Pitkeathley argued at that time that these areas of conflict have the potential to stand in the way of better recognition of carers and result in carers being a difficult group to identify. Many of the issues that Pitkeathley was grappling with at the time remain unresolved today and her observation that the change that should have been brought about through legislation required changes at a wider, societal level is apposite. Campaigners and supporters of new legislation and policies point optimistically to their potential to be a game-changer but often are disappointed by the consequences. According to Means et al (2003), the financial and organisational problems that were already entrenched in a creaking system when the National Health Service (NHS) and Community Care Act was passed in 1990 prevented its successful implementation. Hard political and economic priorities easily eclipse the warmth of the rhetoric of family, community and care, even though the *need* for change in the system of care and support is widely accepted. Almost half of the period since 1990 has been spent under austerity policies, which have taken financial stringency to new levels, with serious implications for unpaid care. A historical perspective on policy making sheds light on the trends surrounding these tensions and conflicts over the past 30 years. One such trend is the ageing of the British population. The perception that growing numbers of older people are *en masse* a threat to society because of their reliance on pensions, health and social care services is the subtext of policies on unpaid care. Another trend is the rise in levels of women's employment and education and a slow shift in attitudes towards women's roles as carers. This has not been straightforward, however, and policies on both paid and unpaid care continue to assume gendered roles, although predictions that the supply of unpaid carers would dry up as women embarked on paid employment in greater numbers have not been realised. Unpaid care is provided *differently* but not less than it was 30 years ago, as is discussed in the next chapter.

The NHS Community Care Act, 1990 is the starting point for the policy analysis in this book. It is fully acknowledged that this starting point is somewhat artificial and that references to unpaid care can be identified in policies in the 1980s. Indeed, as the discussion in Chapter 2 demonstrates, interest in developing knowledge about unpaid care had already been stimulated and data-gathering had begun. It was, however, the 1990 Act that established the marketised form of social care, which has had significant implications for unpaid care and carers. It was a key stage in the development of the tense and often troubled relationship between 'formal' services and unpaid care. The policy agenda of care in the community is discussed next to set the scene for the analysis that follows through the book.

Care in the community, care by the community

Pressure to shut down the institutions housing older and disabled people and people with mental health problems reached a crescendo in the 1980s, having been building over decades before. The pace of change was a cause of disquiet among policy commentators. Walker, for example, argued that the 'history of community care policies in Britain is one of painfully slow progress towards timid goals' (Walker 1982: 16). During the 1980s, ideas about non-institutional forms of care generated intense debate about the nature of care and who should take responsibility for its provision, as analysed by Baldwin and Twigg (1991). Care at home was contrasted with institutional care in unqualified positive terms, except that at the time feminist commentators questioned who was doing the caring and at what cost. Hilary Land (1978) had already observed that most, if not all, social policies assumed a gendered division of labour within families and that those who had no family to care for them were prioritised for home (domiciliary) care services. The argument was, therefore, that care in the community, as it came to be known, *reinforced* the perceived 'natural' association between women and care, as home was understood as the domain of women, whose activities encompassed not only housework but also the care of children and relatives that needed support; activities that were referred to by Graham (1983) as 'a labour of love'. Nevertheless, policy makers presented the home as the preferred place of care unproblematically. Indeed, Glendinning (1986: 200) commented that 'the increasing visibility of and explicit reliance upon relatives and friends to provide day to day physical and social care' was *the* major policy development of the time. In 1981, the White Paper *Growing Older* stated that the 'primary sources of support and care for elderly people are informal and voluntary' and that care *in* the community 'must increasingly mean *by* the community'. The role of public authorities, as set out in the White Paper, was to sustain and develop – but never displace – such support and care (DHSS 1981: 3). The development of non-institutionalised forms of care represented both the success of campaigns to end the pernicious effects of institutionalisation on older and disabled people *and* the opportunity to develop a mixed economy of welfare in place of the largely state-run system. It was during the 1980s that the British form of a mixed economy developed, in which statutory, voluntary and private (for-profit) providers all became involved in the provision of social care, including residential and domiciliary services.

At the same time, a conflict emerged between the disability rights movement and the carers' movement. The Disabled Persons (Services, Consultation and Representation) Act 1986 had introduced the term 'carer' to British legislation in section 8, which stipulated that when deciding what care services should be provided to a disabled person, a local authority should take account of the ability of the carer to continue to provide care on a regular basis. Cook (2007) maintains that during the passage of this legislation, carers' groups wanted stronger wording to support carers' rights, while the groups representing disabled people were concerned not to shift the emphasis of the policy away from its primary purpose of supporting disabled people. Extracts from the Report of the House of Commons Social Services Committee (House of Commons 1990) give an indication of these tensions. On behalf of the British Council of Organisations of Disabled People, Richard Wood, the Director, said:

> It worries me when I hear this word 'care'. The fact that the Government paper 'Caring for People' has 'caring' in its title worries me intensely because many, many disabled people do not need caring for, but they are people who are entitled to benefits and they are people who need basic services in order to lead full and independent lives. (House of Commons 1990: paragraph 7)

In response to this point, the Committee undertook to be mindful about terminology, especially in their references to dependency, but insisted that their report was about community care from the perspective of carers of those disabled people who *are* dependent on their carer because of the severity of their conditions: 'It is impossible to exaggerate the burden placed on a carer of a relative or friend who is severely disabled, frail, demented or elderly or all four' (House of Commons 1990: paragraph 9). These conflicting views re-emerge throughout the period under discussion in this book and are examined in greater depth in Chapters 2 and 6. Importantly, what became a bitter dispute between, on the one hand, feminist critiques of unpaid care and, on the other, disabled people who rejected the idea of care has given rise to new perspectives, also examined in greater depth.

At this time, an underlying assumption among policy makers was that in community care the private sector would be more efficient and consumer-oriented than the statutory sector. Although privately owned and run residential care homes had been part of the social care system from the outset they were not major players. The aim was to reduce statutory provision and promote the private sector and the balance between statutory and private provision began to reverse. A key strategy of the Conservative government was to provide funding for residents in private sector care homes through the social security system. This provided the owners with a steady guaranteed source of revenue and attracted more people to become owners of care homes. It became increasingly evident, however, that this funding strategy was ruinously expensive. In addition, it had a perverse effect on *community* care policies because local authorities could save money by placing people in private care homes instead of developing domiciliary services in people's own homes. Action was necessary to sort out the funding and organisation of care in the community and the government set up a review, led by Roy Griffiths, with an advisory group that included Jill Pitkeathley in her capacity as director of the Carers National Association. The report of this review body, *Community Care: An Agenda for Action*, published in 1988, made this statement:

> Families, friends, neighbours and other local people provide the majority of care in response to needs, which they are uniquely well placed to identify and respond to. ... The proposals take as their starting point that this is as it should be, and the first task of publicly provided services is to support and where possible strengthen these networks of carers. (Griffiths 1988: 5)

The subsequent White Paper, *Caring for People* (DH 1989), took up many of the recommendations in the Griffiths Report and the NHS Community Care Act 1990 (NHSCC Act) was passed into legislation. This Act was a landmark in social care policies and practices. Its emphasis on enabling people to remain in their own homes or in homely environments was linked with the development of the mixed economy of welfare. The role of statutory agencies as providers continued to be reduced while the roles of the private (for-profit) and the voluntary (not-for-profit) sectors were increased. The Act introduced a clear separation between the process of needs assessment (local authorities) and the provision of services to meet assessed needs (mainly private and voluntary agencies). The mechanism through which this was arranged was care management, described at the time as the cornerstone of high-quality care (DH 1990). Care management changed the nature of professional social work practice with adult service users, as discussed further in Chapter 5. It was envisaged that when care managers assessed individuals' needs, they would plan services in partnership with service users, to produce a 'tailor-made' package of care. It was also envisaged that in the assessment and care planning processes carers would be consulted and their needs taken into account. The concept of 'tailor-made' contrasted with institutionalised forms of care and was a forerunner of subsequent ideas about personalised care, also discussed in Chapter 5. The concept of a 'package of care' was a novel way of describing services and presented care as a commodity that could be packaged, purchased and provided, with provision being more varied and centred upon the particular preferences of service users. It follows that it was care as an *activity* (caring for) that became the dominant theme within publicly funded services, while care as a *relationship* (caring about) remained a private, family matter and attention to the needs and rights of unpaid carers, although promised in the Griffiths Report, was overlooked in the legislation.

Enabling people to remain in their own homes or in care homes that were as homely as possible has remained a fundamental principle of statutory health and social care services to this day. In recognition of this, one of six key objectives of the White Paper *Caring for People* (DH 1989) was to make support for carers a high priority. As already discussed, this objective was never satisfactorily met in the legislation and carers found themselves with additional pressures arising from the new system of care and overlooked during service users' needs assessments. This was unsurprising, given the waning of interest in unpaid carers through the process of legislation. Indeed, the Practice Guidance on the NHSCC Act 1990 stated that in the event of differences between carers and those they supported more weight should be given to the service users' views (SSI/SWSG 1991).

The unsustainable system of funding private sector care home places through the social security budget was addressed by shifting the budget for residential care to local authorities as a capped block grant, 85 per cent of which was to be spent in the non-statutory sectors. This measure stemmed the unsustainable cost of residential care and removed the incentive to place people in residential care to avoid spending on domiciliary services but it came at a massive cost to unpaid carers. There were no new resources to support the policy, despite rising demand for domiciliary services. Consequently, local authority managers' room for manoeuvre was extremely limited and they prioritised those service users that they perceived to be in greatest need, which in general meant those that had no carer.

It bears repetition that the inadequacy of resources for community care in local authorities was not a by-product of challenging economic times but the intended outcome of policies to reduce the sphere of activity and influence of the public sector and of local authorities. It was an element of a much wider squeeze on public spending, which left local authorities with the difficult task of developing more (and more innovative) services but with fewer resources to cover the cost and less autonomy in deciding how to spend their money. This created major headaches for social services managers who were given additional responsibility for managing the finances and implementing increasingly stringent eligibility criteria. As Parsloe commented at the time:

> The NHS & Community Care Act backs a whole field of horses, with the two front-runners being user choice and scarce resources. Local authorities are apparently expected to give equal weight to empowering users and keeping within their own budget. None of the official guidance even recognises the conflict, let alone shows how these two competing aims are to be balanced. (Parsloe 1993: 16–17)

The negative impact of a lack of statutory arrangements for unpaid carers was foreseen by many organisations and groups. During their discussions on the 1989 White Paper *Caring for People*, the House of Commons Social Services Committee had received evidence from a range of organisations, including this from a director of social services:

> The core of the White Paper proposals is not just to shift care from residential to non-residential but to shift from public-funded provision to family care ... what should be of concern is the clear existing unmet need among carers. Leaving aside the issue of who should provide public-funded care, the need for additional public funded services should be evident. (House of Commons Social Services Committee 1990: para 100)

The then Minister for Health, Virginia Bottomley, argued that the lack of specific statutory measures for carers was not a problem, because Practice Guidance, *Getting it Right for Carers* (DH 1991), emphasised the importance of ensuring that services were designed to meet carers' needs – as defined by carers – as well as ensuring that carers were well informed about their entitlements. Others were less sanguine, emphasising the need for properly costed services, such as respite care, specialist support for service users, help for carers to remain in work and a more comprehensive system of benefits.

Evidence on the outcomes of the NHSCC Act proved the sceptics right (Parker 1999). The more concentrated focus on people in greatest need enabled more people who would otherwise have been admitted to a care home to remain in their own homes. This can be regarded as a policy success but at the same time this more concentrated focus led to increased reliance on families to fill the gaps for those who were no longer perceived to be a priority. In addition, the focus on those in greatest need skewed services towards personal care, which reduced the availability of practical help. Instead of increasing choice, therefore, the emphasis on targeting those in greatest need *curtailed* choice for service users and carers and drew attention away from the preventive capacity of social care. Parker (1999) pointed out that the Practice Guidance on the NHSCC Act, 1990, had been that priority should be based not on the basis of levels of disability but on the capacity of the individual and their carers to manage needs. A national inspection of local authority support for carers between 1994 and 1995 highlighted the tendency to prioritise individuals without an unpaid carer and found that home care services had ceased to be involved in cleaning and practical help and became focused on personal care in a way that was 'not always helpful to carers' (SSI 1995: 41). Evidently, the central role of carers in the production of the Griffiths Report had not led to the desired aims in the legislation.

At the same time, the organisational changes brought about by the reforms and the establishment of the mixed economy led to a complex system of provision that was difficult for service users and carers to understand and negotiate. For adults with mental health problems a parallel policy, the Care Programme Approach, was established in 1991. This caused confusion in the early years and according to Heron (1998) was somewhat removed from mainstream carer activity. For example, Heron noted the use of the term 'family' in the context of mental health where the word 'carer' was applied in the context of old age or disability. As Mandelstam (1999: 27) argued, community care was rife with uncertainties that became an integral part of the system and were exacerbated by the pressure on resources. For example, there was a lack of precision in the meaning of key terms, such as 'need'; a lack of clarity about what constituted a 'duty' on the part of local authorities or 'powers' that they might choose to exercise. Walker (1994: 11) described the state of community care for older people after 1990 as a nightmare in which family carers were 'driven to the end of their endurance by the need to provide 24-hour care to a spouse or parent'. Research by the Carers National Association found that four out of five carers believed their circumstances had either remained the same or deteriorated since the introduction of community care (Warner 1995). Apparently, the claim of the Minister for Health in her statement to the Social Services Committee in 1990 was, as feared, wrong.

The NHSCC Act applied in England, Scotland and Wales. In Northern Ireland the White Paper *People First: Community Care in Northern Ireland in the 1990s* (DHSS 1991), set out how community care would be implemented in the four integrated Health and Social Services Boards. The Northern Ireland community care arrangements had some advantages over those in the other three administrations because more resources were available to set up community-based alternatives to institutional services. In addition, the integrated system of health and social care meant there were fewer disputes over which agency was responsible for funding services. As far as carers were concerned, however, the introduction of community care in Northern Ireland was a disappointment. Tonks (1994) argued that because the energies of the Boards were focused on their reorganisation into Trusts, carers remained ignorant about their rights under the new system. In addition, the closure of long-stay hospitals reduced the availability of respite services. Underpinning the Northern Ireland *People First* White Paper was a clear philosophy on unpaid care: 'the obligations of kin and affection will remain powerful motivators. It is in society's interest to sustain that motivation and to see that appropriate packages of support are assembled for people who are able and willing to care for others' (DHSS 1991). The philosophy encapsulated in this statement was and remains a strong motivator for policy makers throughout the UK. That is, support for carers is needed because it is in the public interest to ensure that their motivation to care is sustained. The impact of the community care legislation on unpaid care was rapid, seen in the additional demands on unpaid carers, as well as in the confusion that surrounded the emerging mixed economy of care. Since these early days of care in the community, the same fundamental political ideology has continued to dominate, as evidenced in policies on restraint in public expenditure on public services, the preference for the private, for-profit sector over the public sector as service provider and the assumption that families should be the main providers of care. Parker and Clark referred to these as the 'unholy trio', which in combination, led inexorably towards greater pressure on unpaid care (Parker and Clarke 2002: 349).

This brief overview of the policy and organisational backdrop to the policies and practices in this book is inevitably incomplete, but the following implications for unpaid care are highlighted as they re-emerge throughout the book. First, unpaid care made care in the community a possibility. The 1989 White Paper, *Caring for People*, recognised the central role of unpaid carers. The subsequent legislation did not refer to carers, however, nor were resources provided to fund support for carers. The gap between the rhetoric and reality of policies on unpaid care was clear from this point on. Second, the implementation of care in the community was patchy and unsatisfactory, which increased uncertainty and complexity within a turbulent social care system. This added to the pressures on unpaid carers and those they supported. Third, in the context of tight resources, carers' needs were unlikely to be at the forefront of providers' attention. On the contrary, their unpaid contributions became a major part of the solution to the problem of meeting need. At the same time, as pointed out, a parallel view of carers emerged as those who were under extreme pressure and in need of policy makers' attention. Fourth, the introduction of care in the community generated tensions and disagreements about the concept of care and the direction of policy in relation to carers and disabled people (Thomas, 1993). The idealisation of care provided within the family, seen in policy statements discussed here, draws attention to the divide between public services and private, family arrangements. While policies emphasised choice in services, which were to be tailor-made to suit the needs of individuals, in practice in unpaid care choice was curtailed, including choice over whether to become a carer at all or to what extent.

The title of the book reflects the intention to develop a critique of policies on unpaid care, those that have been about unpaid carers being the main interest. There is no intention to deny the pressures that unpaid carers experience or the continued tendency by professionals in the care system to take them for granted or the potential of policies to improve the lives of individuals in care relationships. The question that is of key interest is what has been achieved by successive policies on support for unpaid carers and what can be learnt from this reflection on the past to inform future decisions and actions.

The organisation of the book

The discussion in the subsequent chapters begins with an outline and discussion of relevant research and key policies and progresses to more critical analysis of these policies in context and to a discussion of broader questions about the nature of dependency and care.

Chapter 2 gives an account of the development of knowledge about unpaid care since the 1980s, exploring the growth of interest in the subject. The discussion includes the ways in which knowledge has been produced, the focus and methods of research and knowledge development as well as the key lessons arising from research. The sheer quantity of research is a matter of interest, and an important element of the discussion is the role of research in shaping ideas about unpaid care and unpaid carers. This chapter also introduces important theoretical developments that have emerged over the same period, including those related to the ethics of care and to disabled people's rights.

In Chapter 3, the focus is on key policies and strategies on unpaid care since the 1990s. These include policies specifically about support for unpaid carers as well as others of particular relevance and importance to this discussion. The focus is on policies in the sphere of social care, although debates and measures related to carers' income and paid employment are also considered. The policies developed in the devolved governments in Scotland, Wales and Northern Ireland are included, not to provide a comparative analysis but to point to notable differences and similarities in aims and outcomes. Key themes arising from the discussion are presented as a basis for the critical analysis in subsequent chapters. The historical perspective highlights continuities and changes in policies on unpaid care in all parts of the UK, key elements of which include the recognition of carers as a distinctive group; shifts in the balance of responsibility for care away from publicly funded provision towards unpaid carers; the increased role of unpaid carers as participants in the policy process and service planning at national and local levels; and tensions between policies on support for unpaid carers and other social care policies.

Chapter 4 picks up on these key themes to examine practices in relation to unpaid care at the local level, and the influence of policies on service provision. Professional perceptions of carers are examined with reference to the model developed by Twigg and Atkin (1994) which categorises these as background resources, co-workers, co-clients and superseded carers. Professional practices in assessment are examined, including a focus on the changing roles of professionals as assessors of need in the context of changing policies on support for carers. The introduction of personalisation and the tensions that arise between the rights of carers and disabled people are key elements of the discussion in this chapter. The period in which policies on unpaid carers have been introduced has been one of organisational tensions, which have had significant implications for professional practice, including the pressures on local authorities to reduce their expenditure at the same time as developing new and innovative practice with carers.

In Chapter 5, theories of the policy process are drawn upon to analyse the gap between the rhetoric and realities of policies on unpaid care. The economic and political contexts of policies are discussed, not only in relation to their hindrance of policy implementation but also in terms of their importance as an overarching political project. The discussion focuses on the recurrence of themes in policies on unpaid care and the framing of unpaid care as an issue for policy in the context of organisational and financial pressures on local authorities. It examines ideas about governance and the role of carers' organisations in local networks and partnerships.

In Chapter 6, the discussion extends to consider the broader ethical and philosophical issues raised by the development of policies on unpaid care. It returns to the observations of Andrew Dilnot concerning the need for governments to have courage and strength of will to develop policies on social care. It questions the purpose and meaning of policies that increase the rights of carers as a specific group within social care, when those rights are regularly quashed by the overarching imperative to reduce public spending. The feminist ethics of care and key critiques of this are discussed. The impacts of neoliberal policies on unpaid care are considered, with reference in particular to the care deficit but also to the development of ideas about care, in the context of increasingly precarious social and economic environments. Potential alternatives to the existing policy trends are examined.

In Chapter 7, the conclusions are drawn from the historical reflection of policies, and their role in shaping experiences of unpaid care in practice. Possible alternative policy approaches are considered, based on a different framing of care and carers. The discussion provides a critique of policies that emphasise a distinctive carer identity and argues for policies based on the alternative paradigm of caring as a widespread and diverse activity that involves us all and of care as a relationship.

A note on terminology

This is an area of study in which terminology is often contested and the unstable nature of definitions is understood. The term 'unpaid carers' is preferred over 'family carers', which does not cover the diversity of caring arrangements, or 'informal carers' which conveys a much more casual picture of unpaid care than is accurate or fair. The term 'carers' is understood to also cover paid care workers and, where necessary, the term 'unpaid carers' is used to avoid misunderstandings. The instability of the 'unpaid' description is accepted, as is the boundary between paid and unpaid care: paid carers often carry out additional work unpaid, while some unpaid carers receive payment through the direct payments scheme or through the Carer's Allowance. The term 'disabled people' is intended to cover people with learning disabilities as well as mental health problems and long-term physical health problems. There are many ways in which the experiences of these groups overlap, not least in terms of the relevance of the social model of disability to their circumstances and the disabling effects of being within the care system.

The discussion is limited to adult carers, who are covered by the relevant legislation from the 1995 Carers (Recognition and Services) Act onwards. Young carers (those aged under 18) are excluded because their needs are covered by a different legislative framework.

An empirical research project is referred to throughout the book, to illustrate points of discussion. *The Impact of the 2014 Care Act on Older Carers of Older People* is referred to as the 'Older Carers' project. References include Lloyd and Jessiman (2017), Jessiman and Lloyd (2018), Lloyd et al (2020) and O'Rourke et al (2021). A subsequent update of part of this project was conducted during the period of the COVID-19 pandemic: 'Online advice to carers: An updated review of local authority websites in England' (Willis et al 2021). Both of these projects were funded by the National Institute for Health and Care Research (NIHR) School for Social Care Research but the opinions expressed are those of the researchers.

2

Research and knowledge development on unpaid care in the UK

Introduction

This chapter examines the ways in which knowledge about unpaid care has developed over the past three decades. An intriguing question is whether patterns of unpaid care have changed or more information is now available, which sheds new light on long-standing patterns. In addressing this question, further questions arise, including *how* has knowledge on unpaid care developed over recent decades and to what end? Such questions matter, not only because knowledge is essential to the development of appropriate support for unpaid care but also because these questions draw attention to the complexities of care and to the way that care is characterised in the policy process. For example, Parker (1990) reflected on the popular illusion that in modern societies the family no longer cares about its members with support needs. Despite copious research evidence to the contrary, this misconception remains influential. For example, in 2013, Jeremy Hunt MP (the then Secretary of State for Health) argued that there was a need to 'reinvigorate the social contract between generations' so that older people in Britain could enjoy similar levels of 'reverence and respect' as their counterparts in Asia (Butler 2013). In 2017, David Mowat MP urged people to accept their duty to look after their elderly parents, not least because of the 'volume of numbers that we see coming down the track' (Asthana 2017). Words such as reverence, respect and duty are heavily freighted with moral overtones, although, arguably, moral standards apply irrespective of the numbers of people involved. David Mowat's statement gives the political context: unpaid care for family members is a hot topic for policy makers *because* of the numbers of people involved.

In 2021, a Family Resources Survey for the Department for Work and Pensions (DWP) estimated that between 2019 and 2020 around 4.5 million people in the UK (around 7 per cent of the population) were providing 'informal' care: that is, where caring is not a paid job (DWP 2021). The survey findings are at odds with those of Carers UK, which estimated that prior to the COVID-19 pandemic there were 'up to 9.1 million carers in the UK' and that this number had increased dramatically by 4.5 million during the course of the pandemic (Carers UK 2020). There is still uncertainty, therefore, about the numbers of unpaid carers in the population and differences in the methods of calculating these. Differences are partly a consequence of sampling methods used by researchers but also how individuals answer research questions related to care and whether they perceive their relationships or their activities as care per se or as part and parcel of ordinary life. The Social Market Foundation (Petrie and Kirkup 2018) argued that accurate and detailed data are necessary to ensure that policy is based upon a realistic expectation of what unpaid carers can do and an understanding of how providing care affects their lives but evidently accuracy is not easy to achieve.

Despite uncertainties over numbers, there is now a better understanding of the diversity of unpaid care than there was three decades ago, including differences between carers in terms of their gender, ethnic background and age as well as the kind of care they provide and the impact of caring on their activities, health and opportunities. More is known now about different kinds of care relationships and changing patterns of care needs. Yet, as research on unpaid care frequently concludes, further questions and issues remain to be examined. Inequalities between unpaid carers related to socioeconomic class and ethnicity, for example, are not well understood. There has been research interest in identifying groups of carers about whom little is known – the so-called 'hidden carers' (see, for example, Willis et al 2011) but particular groups remain poorly understood. A historical perspective illuminates not only the past but also the present by highlighting the gaps, changes and continuities in the relationship between research and policy making.

Since the 1960s carers' organisations have played a major part in promoting interest in unpaid care, exposing the challenges and injustices faced by unpaid carers and generating evidence to support their claims and demands (Kohner 1993). Their campaigning and research have been revelatory, bringing into the public domain what was by tradition a private activity. A criticism sometimes levelled at this research was that carers' organisations tended to represent their membership, rather than carers more broadly. Olsen et al (1997), for example, examined the involvement of carers' groups in local policy development and pointed to the lack of carers from minority ethnic groups. Nevertheless, the evidence produced by carers' organisations has shed light on daily experiences of caring and the many impacts of caring on carers' health, finances and career opportunities. The specific challenges for carers brought about by the COVID-19 pandemic drew attention to pre-existing weaknesses in the social care system. It was significant that from the early days of the pandemic, family carers were frequently overlooked in terms of publicly funded support, but carers' organisations were quick to gather evidence to highlight these difficulties as well as to provide a crucially important information resource for carers and local authorities (Carers UK 2020).

Taking the long view: the development of knowledge about unpaid care and caring

It was through research in the 1980s that the term 'carer' emerged in policy documents, having been used from around 1980 by the then National Council for the Single Woman and her Dependants (Cook 2007). According to Bytheway and Johnson (1998), the emergence of the term 'carer' was a consequence of the sampling strategies used by researchers in projects concerning older people's use of community care services. 'Principal carers' of older service users became research participants and their experiences featured in the data gathering. Bytheway and Johnson (1998) pointed out that because there was a particular interest in identifying the effects of shortages of formal services, it was considered appropriate to refer to carers as a discrete group. The consequence, however, was to limit knowledge of unpaid care to situations where service users were already known to social services. At this point, therefore, carers were defined as another category in the system of community care. The circumstances of carers more generally were not investigated and, as a result, policy makers perceived carers only in terms of their family relationships to those already known to service providers. This narrow perspective meant, for example, that the role of gay men caring for their partners and friends with HIV through the 1980s and 1990s was almost completely overlooked in policy debates on unpaid care (Rosenfeld et al 2012).

Arber and Ginn (1990) suggested that the term 'carer' was born out of feminist writing on the domestic labour of women. Following Land (1978), Finch and Groves (1983) argued that the term 'community' was a euphemism for care provided by women. They argued that the cultural definition of women as 'carers' was part of wider assumptions about the sexual division of labour, which influenced women's life chances and maintained their social and economic disadvantage. This, together with other papers in social policy journals, stimulated feminist critiques of community care through the 1980s, the key points of which were summarised by Baldwin and Twigg (1991) as follows:

- that the care of non-spousal dependent people falls primarily to women;
- that it is unshared to a significant extent by relatives or by statutory or voluntary agencies;
- that it creates burdens and material costs, which are a source of significant inequalities between men and women;
- that many women nevertheless accept the role of informal carer and, indeed, derive satisfaction from doing so; and
- that the reasons for this state of affairs are deeply bound up with the construction of female and male identity, a possibly also with culturally

defined rules about gender-appropriate behaviours. (Baldwin and Twigg 1991: 124)

Baldwin and Twigg (1991) also made the pertinent point that the feminist debate had largely overlooked the common interests shared by carers and those they support. Indeed, they claimed it ignored the impact of being cast as 'dependants' upon those who needed support. They argued that it was possible for community care policies to benefit people with support needs *and* unpaid carers. To achieve this, they suggested, the balance of responsibility should be tilted towards collective, public provision and away from families. In this way, the individual rights of carers and those with support needs could be recognised, giving them greater choice and enhancing respect for disabled people as well as unpaid carers. The fundamentals of the debates that took place in the 1980s are still evident, currently. In 2019, for example, a paper by Carers UK commented that 'caring is often thought of as being part and parcel of a woman's life' (Carers UK 2019b: 2) and that 'women are more likely [than men] to have given up work as a result of caring' (Carers UK 2019b: 3). It also argues that caring should be made more visible and that more public social care services for older and disabled people are needed as well as fairer financial support for carers (Carers UK 2019b).

In 1985, the then annual General Household Survey (GHS) carried out by the Office of Population Census and Surveys included a survey on Informal Carers (Green 1988). This was the first attempt to collect official information on unpaid care. The survey counted as carers those people 'who were looking after, or providing some regular service for, a sick, handicapped or elderly person living in their own or in another household' (Green 1988: 1). It found that there were about 6 million carers in Great Britain, representing one adult in seven (14 per cent of the adult population), with 1.4 million (3 per cent of adults) providing care for 20 hours a week or more. It also found that the peak age for caring was between 45 and 64, that women outnumbered men as carers (3.5 million compared with 2.5 million) and that carers were found equally between different social groups and levels of educational qualification. Single women in the 45–64 age group were found to be more than twice as likely as men or ever-married women to be caring for at least 20 hours per week but this difference did not appear in any other age groups and, overall, single women represented just 11 per cent of all female carers. This was a surprising finding because the view that single women were the predominant group among carers was deeply rooted (Arber and Gilbert 1989). After all, it was the actions of the National Council for the Single Woman and Her Dependants, formed in 1965, which gave rise to the carers' movement (Kohner 1993). To even greater surprise, the survey identified men as constituting 40 per cent of unpaid carers.

Arber and Ginn (1990) reanalysed the findings from this survey to examine more closely the concept of caring itself as well as the stereotype of the 'carer' as a middle-aged woman. The question of what constituted a 'carer' was unclear and, as Arber and Ginn's (1990) analysis showed, the question of self-identification contributed to this lack of clarity. The figure of 6 million carers generated by the survey reflected what they termed a 'maximalist' definition of carer. It included forms of practical support (gardening and shopping, for example) with no lower threshold on the length of time spent on these tasks. Arber and Ginn concluded that because men were more likely to define such occasional practical help as 'care' they would have answered the survey questions differently from women, who would be more likely to regard such help as part of their normal roles within the household. They also queried why policy makers were demanding statistical evidence on unpaid care *at this point in time* and concluded that it was because of simplistic assumptions about demographic trends, including the likely increased demand for care arising from an ageing population on the one hand and a decline in the proportion of middle-aged women in the population on the other. Nevertheless, despite these limitations, Arber and Ginn regarded the 1985 GHS survey as a landmark, since it was the first official recognition that 'domestic labour' made an essential contribution to the community (Arber and Ginn 1990: 431). It raised many questions about what tasks were being carried out, how much time was spent on them, how regularly and frequently, and who had responsibility for ensuring that the care was provided. Crucially, the 1985 GHS survey introduced a distinction between 'caring' as an activity and 'normal support' given within families. Arber and Ginn (1990) argued that a distinction should also be drawn between co-resident and extra-resident care, because although the evidence showed that almost three-quarters of carers supported someone in a separate household, almost three-quarters of the total time spent caring was within co-resident care. Moreover, they pointed out, the bulk of support from statutory services was directed at people without a co-resident carer, meaning that those with the heaviest load (which included a lot of older carers) were the least well supported.

Focused also on the GHSs (including those in 1985 and 1990), Parker and Lawton (1994) developed a typology of unpaid care which was based on the number of people *being helped* rather than on the number of people providing care. This, they argued, provided a more accurate picture of unpaid care, because it took account of individuals who cared for more than one person and showed more about the different ways in which people were helped. They found that of the 1.5 million people caring for 20 or more hours per week, half were caring for more than 50 hours per week. Moreover, these highly involved carers were providing many different types of care. In their typology, *personal* care was the term given to helping adults of all ages with bathing, dressing and using the toilet; *physical* help referred to help with walking and getting in and out of bed; *practical* help included assistance with preparing meals, shopping and housework; *other help* included taking a person out and helping them with paperwork and finances. These categories overlapped in different ways and helped to identify those individuals involved in more substantial levels of caring, involving long hours, often over long periods of time and often in the same household. This group represented about 12 per cent of those who self-identified as carers in the 1985 GHS. It might have been expected that their findings would be taken up by local authorities across the board, with a view to prioritising carers at the 'heavy end' of the spectrum, but Parker and Lawton (1994: 89) found that a 'hierarchy of service substitution' existed, with a bias against people with co-resident carers. They also argued that the community care reforms introduced in the NHS and Community Care Act, 1990 should have been a means of encouraging low-level help as well as providing support to or substituting for those providing substantial care (Parker and Lawton 1994). In making this observation, Parker and Lawton identified an issue that beset social services in subsequent years: how to maintain a broad focus on and provide preventive support for unpaid care *as well as* prioritising those in greatest need, as successive social care policies have demanded.

At the time, Jill Pitkeathley, the director of the Carers National Association argued that a lot more people provided care than the GHS had identified and that the lives of those who cared for fewer hours per week were also, as she expressed it, restricted (Pitkeathley 1989). As Bytheway and Johnson (1998) pointed out, however, Pitkeathley was aware that not all 6 million carers identified in the GHS were spending a large proportion of their time providing physical and personal care. Instead, they argued, her estimate should be understood in the context of her primary aim, which was to build the carers' movement rather than assist local authorities to set priorities for spending on services. Bytheway and Johnson also pointed to the categorisation of Alzheimer's as a disease entity, distinct from 'normal' ageing, which they argued assisted the carers' cause by giving voice to their experiences of caring for people with dementia as distinct from 'normal' family life. This debate reflects how the calculation of numbers of carers in the population mattered in different ways, according to context. The question of how, and to what end, carers are identified recurs throughout this text, as a tension can be identified between the broad picture of numerous and diverse people involved in many types of unpaid care, on the one hand,

and the specific categorisation of a group of carers who qualify for support, on the other.

Patterns and trends in unpaid care

In this section, the focus is on the patterns of and trends in unpaid care and how knowledge about these has developed over the last three decades. Two points need to be borne in mind. First, the population of carers changes over time, due largely to the natural course of population turnover but also, as discussed, to variations in how carers are counted and what counts as caring. Local policies and practices influence the identification of carers: for example, older and disabled carers might not be classified as carers because they are also service users. In addition, caring occurs in dynamic relationships that change over time as people's circumstances change, and these changes affect official recognition of their caring role and their eligibility for services and support.

The shift from institution-based care to community care was, as argued, the major policy influence on patterns and intensity of unpaid care and it established the position of unpaid carers within the social care system, as from the outset the policy of care in the community became care *by* the community. It became normal practice in local authorities to expect families to take on increasing amounts of support and care. Hirst (2001) analysed data from the annual British Household Panel Surveys between 1991 and 1998 and identified an intensification of unpaid caring with increased levels of activities at the 'heavy end' of caring (meaning longer hours and more personal care) and a commensurate decrease at the less demanding end of the spectrum. Associated with this were an increase in co-resident care and in the numbers of individuals caring for one person only. The most striking change Hirst noted was the increase in spouse-caring by men by 8 per cent per year, which was twice the rate of increase in female spouse care. At the same time, women continued to provide the bulk of care overall. This included co-resident care for spouses and disabled children but also intensive support for people in separate households, typically parents and parents-in-law. As Hirst noted, the trend away from multi-generational households occurring during the latter part of the 20th century did not mean a decrease in care; it meant a change in the type of care provided as more older people continued to live in their own homes.

Maher and Green (2002) analysed the data on unpaid care from the GHS conducted every five years from 1985 to 2000. They also identified that over the previous decade there had been little change in the prevalence of caring. In 2000, the data showed there were 6.8 million carers aged 16 and over in Great Britain, or around 16 per cent of the population, up from 14 per cent in 1985. Like Hirst (2001), they found that women were most likely to be involved at the heavy end of caring (11 per cent of women compared with 7 per cent of men); were more likely to care for someone in a separate household (12 per cent compared with 9 per cent); and were more likely to be the main support for the person cared for, whether they were the sole carer or shared the care with a man. Those caring for someone in the same household were more likely to be at the heavy end of caring and one in ten carers spent more than 50 hours per week on their caring responsibilities.

When the Labour government published its Strategy for Carers in 1999 (discussed further in Chapter 3), it drew on the figures in the 1995 GHS. In this Strategy it was estimated that one in six households in Britain contained a carer, which amounted to 5.7 million carers with an additional 250,000 in Northern Ireland. It was recognised that the GHS did not provide the definitive picture of carers and that better knowledge was needed about unpaid care in minority Black and ethnic groups as well as among children and young people. The overall picture of carers at that time was that 58 per cent were women, that they were concentrated in the 45–64 age group, comprising a fifth of all adults in that age group, and that the majority were looking after someone in a separate household. Of the 1.9 million people caring for someone in the same household, over half were caring for their spouses and one-fifth were caring for their disabled or sick children. Unsurprisingly, those providing care for someone in the same household were also caring for the greatest number of hours, with 38 per cent providing more than 50 hours per week. The strategy noted how social trends, such as the increasing number of women in full-time employment, might affect the supply of unpaid care. Indeed, the figures from the GHS demonstrated that women in paid employment were less likely to provide unpaid care. Nevertheless, around two-thirds of carers below the state pension age were in paid employment, or self-employed, and this figure drew attention to the needs of carers who were combining unpaid care with paid work. Increased life expectancy in older age was also identified as a likely cause of increased demand for care and it was noted that there was an increase between 1985 and 1995 in numbers of older people living in the community who were unable to wash themselves or do their household shopping. At the same time, increased life expectancy also generated more spouse care in later life (HM Govt 1999a).

The 2001 Census question on unpaid care

The need for more comprehensive information about unpaid care generated the decision to include a question in the 2001 Census to capture the number of carers and the number of hours spent by each carer on caring activities. A particular emphasis was placed on the need for personal care, indicating growing concern at the time about the perceived cost to public finances of increasing proportions of older people in the UK population. Census question 12 was: 'Do you look after, or give any help or support to family members, friends, neighbours or others because of long-term physical or mental ill-health or disability or problems related to old age?' This was followed up with questions about the time individuals spent caring in a typical week:

- 1–19 hours
- 20–49 hours
- over 50 hours

In addition to the question concerning care giving, an additional question (Census question 13) asked: 'Do you have a long-term illness, health problem or disability which limits your daily activity or the work you can do?' This combination of questions was intended to identify if the person cared for was in the same household as the carer but did not identify if an individual lived with someone who was disabled while also caring for a different person in another household. The 2001 Census estimated that there were 5.9 million adults in Britain looking after a relative or friend in need of support because of age or frailty, physical or learning disability or illness. Of these, 56 per cent (3.3 million people) were in good health, compared with 70 per cent of those who provide no unpaid care (see Doran et al 2003). Analysis by Young et al (2006) clarified this point by comparing the data from the Census with that provided by the GHS. Using both sets of data they highlighted variations along geographical, socioeconomic and ethnic lines. In areas of deprivation, a higher proportion of people were unpaid carers and individual disadvantage was associated with being a carer. Local authorities with the highest proportion of the population providing 20 or more hours per week of unpaid care included Neath Port Talbot and Merthyr Tydfil in Wales; Easington in the North East; and Barking and Dagenham, Tower Hamlets and Newham in London. This pattern was evidence of a link between socioeconomic status and unpaid care. At the same time, the likelihood of providing unpaid care for more than 20 hours a week was significantly greater in the Bangladeshi and Pakistani communities – twice as likely as the White population – even when socioeconomic status was accounted for.

Dahlberg et al (2007) also analysed data from the 2001 Census and showed that among the population of the UK aged under 70, women were more likely to become carers (11.3 per cent compared to 8.6 per cent of men) and that they were likely to be caring for more hours. After the age of 70, however, this pattern was reversed. A further finding from their analysis was that, although unpaid care was most common in the 45–59 age group, carers aged 70 and over spent more time caring. Del Bono et al (2009), however, pointed to the effect of marital or partnership status on the likelihood of being a carer to argue that once this was accounted for, women were more likely to be carers at any age.

The 2001 Census generated a great deal of interest and analysis as data identified new information. It also raised new questions for research, notably, the impact of caring on carers' health, opportunities and working lives. The 2011 Census showed that the number of carers had grown by 600,000, with the greatest increase being among those who cared for 50 or more hours per week. The increase in unpaid care was evident across almost all local authorities but geographical differences remained – more than twice as many people in Neath Port Talbot provided unpaid care as in the London Borough of Wandsworth (14.6 per cent compared to 6.5 per cent). In fact, the percentage figures for the whole of Wales were higher than England (just over 12 per cent compared to just over 10 per cent) with only those at the lower end of intensity being comparable. Within England, the regions with the highest proportion of the population providing unpaid care were the North West, North East and Midlands (ONS 2013). Jepson (2020) pointed to figures from the Scottish Census that estimated that there were between 700,000 and 800,000 unpaid carers in Scotland, of whom 29,000 were aged under the age of 18. They also drew on analysis published by Carers UK (Zhang et al 2019), which indicated that between 1991 and 2018, 65 per cent of adults in Scotland have been an unpaid carer and that on average a Scottish person has a 50:50 chance of becoming a carer by the age of 49.

Analysis conducted in 2018 by the Social Market Foundation (Petrie and Kirkup 2018) estimated that between 2015 and 2017, there were 7.6 million family carers over the age of 16 in the UK (14.5 per cent of the population aged 16 and over). They also calculated that there had been an increase of half a million in the number of carers over the previous decade and an increase in the hours of care provided, with 28 per cent providing 20 hours per week or more in 2015 compared with 24 per cent in 2005. The number of hours an individual spends in providing care is a widely accepted indicator of intensity of caring but Petrie and Kirkup (2018) also point to the *kind* of help provided, noting that of those adults who provided care to their parents in 2015, 19 per cent were supporting them with personal care tasks, such as bathing, getting dressed and eating, referred to as Activities of Daily Living. This compared to 16 per cent in 2005 (Petrie and Kirkup 2018: 4). It is noteworthy, also, that the category of those caring for '50 hours or more per week' used in the Census is unsatisfactory, as it includes some who are caring for 100 hours per week or more.

The increasing numbers of unpaid carers are revealing not only about demographic trends but also about policy decisions and changes in patterns of provision of formal care. The increase in care between spouses, for example, reflects not only the ageing of the population and changes in patterns of women's employment but also the reduction in formal care services. The perceived cost of an ageing population provided politicians with a rationale for a reduction in the provision of services on the grounds that maintaining services at the current level was unaffordable. Projected increases in numbers of people in the oldest age groups added a sense of urgency, as the earlier quote from David Mowat MP indicated (Asthana 2017). The increasing numbers of unpaid carers is inextricably linked with reductions in publicly funded practical support in the home as well as the increased concentration of services on lower numbers of people with more intensive needs. Post-1990, formal support was unavailable to those who would have been considered eligible for 'home help' services prior to 1990, leaving unpaid carers to pick up the responsibility for practical help. Modelling by Pickard et al (2000) suggested that services for older people should be provided on a 'carer-blind' basis, so that there would be no assumptions made about what a carer might be able to do. They also identified that, contrary to common opinion, this would not be too costly to implement, a point that indicates that despite calls at that time for evidence of 'what works', policy makers had other agendas and priorities to consider.

Debates and disputes in research

Nolan et al (1996) questioned whether the already voluminous literature on family caregiving meant that the subject had already been 'done to death'. They could not have imagined then the quantity of research that would be conducted in subsequent years. They also pointed to the influence of research activity on how family care was perceived, arguing that much of what had been written had been dominated by specific theoretical perspectives and methodological stances. They singled out the strong feminist strand of writing, including that by Finch and Groves (1983) and Dalley (1983), which, they argued, had limited perceptions of family care. They pointed to four main themes in this literature:

- a predominant focus on the burdens of caring;
- a concentration on the tasks of caring;
- a static view of care relationships, arising from quantitative cross-sectional studies; and
- a focus on the caregiver rather than the cared-for person.

Nolan et al (1996) perceived a need for a fuller, more nuanced picture of caring in all its complexities and diversity. They argued that attention should be paid to relatively neglected areas, such as the potential for satisfaction and positive experiences of caring. They also called for greater attention to the ways in which carers manage their situations to identify practical lessons from experience that could benefit other carers and those they support. They acknowledged that there were good reasons to develop policy for carers as a group, since carers shared sufficient needs in common, but they called for a more coherent and empirically tested account of unpaid care that would inform policy makers and help to ensure sensitivity to the diversity of caring relationships. Their point about the diversity of caring is important. Research in the 1980s and 1990s was amassing a great deal of quantitative data about unpaid care but not about its diversity. There were, for example, large gaps in knowledge about unpaid care among minority Black and ethnic groups and among partners and friends of people with HIV-related illness (Carlisle 2000). The GHS, which spawned a great deal of feminist research, had not asked about the ethnic backgrounds of respondents (Boushel 2000). Cook (2007) identified the lack of representation of minority Black and ethnic carers in the Carers National Association as well as the slow response of the Association to their own staff members' concerns about this as one of the carers' movement's historical mistakes.

As discussed, knowledge development about unpaid care has been strongly influenced by the carers' movement, through their publicisation of the circumstances of unpaid carers. It is the action of carers' groups over three decades, the two known today as Carers UK and the Carers Trust being the most influential, that have distinguished unpaid carers as a group with diverse needs and circumstances but with sufficient characteristics and experiences in common to be recognisable within the population in general and the social care system in particular. In their campaigning work in the 1990s they not only asserted the justice of their case for recognition but also provided data about the circumstances of carers and the impact of caring on them. Their findings have been a noteworthy feature of the changing landscape of information about carers over the period in question. The annual surveys conducted by Carers UK have been a key element of this, providing empirical evidence, raising awareness and justifying their claims for better support, including evidence of the economic value of unpaid care (Buckner and Yeandle 2007, 2015).

From the early 1990s, disabled activists, theorists and researchers objected strongly to the feminist research of the time, and rejected the term 'care' (Morris 1993). In Morris' view, feminist researchers had demonstrated an inability to identify with the subjective experiences of disabled people and had therefore forfeited the right to comment on the best arrangements for meeting disabled people's requirements. Thomas (2007) traced this dispute through British academic publications, in which some feminist theorists suggested that the best alternative to the exploitation of women as unpaid carers was the development of new forms of residential living arrangements. Unsurprisingly, after the success of campaigns to close institutions, this suggestion was fiercely opposed by disabled people. Thomas (2007) commented that much soul-searching went on among feminist researchers, with the result that research was conducted with greater attention to the perspectives of both care providers and recipients, including that by Parker (1993), Twigg (1992, 2000) and Parker and Clarke (2002).

From within the disability rights movement, Watson et al (2004) sought a way forward out of the strife that had developed and focused on points of common interest between the sides. They noted that the combination of campaigning and academic research in both feminist and disability movements was not unproblematic, as the research was based on particular stances and, as they noted, research cannot always capture the 'hopes, ambitions, desires and sorrows' of people (Watson et al 2004: 339). In addition, they argued that the priority given to disabled people's control over the provision of help does not adequately account for the interpersonal relationships involved in care but sets up 'a mechanical relationship in which intimacy is eclipsed'. A further point raised was that the development of direct payments as a way forward for disabled people to be in control of their own support needs often resulted in the exploitation of personal assistants as low-paid personal assistants. This, Watson et al argued, should be rejected on the grounds that the liberation of one set of oppressed people should not be at the expense of another. Moreover, both feminist and disability activists critiqued the promotion of 'independence' as a means of emancipation. For feminists, the independence of disabled and older people had come at their expense, while many disabled people also resisted the pressure to be 'independent', when it was a means of forcing them to fit in with the norms of an able-bodied society. Watson et al (2004) proposed that, instead, the focus should be on interdependence, through careful analysis of the ways in which people negotiate their way through the daily challenges of caring and employment, how these are restricted, and how they can become routinised in gendered ways. The idea of interdependence raises deep philosophical questions about human relationships but also poses a challenge in terms of its application in policy and practice, as is discussed in subsequent chapters in this book.

The feminist ethics of care and its critics

The has been a wide diversity of feminist research on care (Fine 2007) and an important school of thought that has emerged over the past four decades is the feminist ethics of care. In what Hankivsky (2005) referred to as the 'first generation' of care theorists, an intense debate occurred during the 1980s, particularly in North America, concerning the relationship between justice and care. Feminist care theorists, such as Gilligan (1993) and Noddings (1984), articulated critiques of liberal theories of justice, such as that developed by Rawls (1971). These critiques focused on the depiction of human autonomy as essentially individualistic and rational, meaning that the purpose of care was to enable the individual who needed it to attain or regain autonomy, independent of a need for care. In contrast, the feminist ethicists' position was that individual human autonomy was not a state of being prior to relationships but could only be achieved *through* relationships and through care.

The second generation of care theorists that followed focused on the ways that justice and care could and should co-exist. In 1991, Berenice Fisher and Joan Tronto published *Towards a Feminist Theory of Care* in which they defined care as 'a species activity that includes everything we do to maintain, continue and repair our "world" so that we can live in it as well as possible. That world includes our bodies, our selves, and our environment, all of which we seek to interweave in a complex, life-sustaining web' (Fisher and Tronto 1991: 40). The term 'everything we do' encapsulates the feminist ethicists' position that care is fundamental to human life because dependency is inherent in the human condition. Fisher and Tronto challenged the perceived boundary between care and justice, as well as that between the private sphere, traditionally seen as the natural site of care, and the public sphere, where political decisions are made about the allocation of resources. Tronto (1993) developed her political ethic of care into a four-phase model that has been adopted widely as a framework for analysis and a basis for conducting research (Brannelly and Barnes 2022). Tronto suggested four interconnected 'phases' of care: caring about; taking care of; caregiving; and care receiving. Caring about refers to attentiveness or noticing a need. The second phase, taking care of, refers to taking responsibility for acting upon that need either directly or through a third party. The motivation for taking care of varies but includes obligation, duty or love. Caregiving, the third phase, relates to the competence and capacities of those who take responsibility, while the fourth phase, care receiving, requires an understanding of care from the standpoint of the person who is being cared for.

The model applies at individual, community or societal levels. Unpaid care remains a largely private sphere activity although policies have brought it into the public sphere. The caregiving element refers not only to the competence of individuals giving care on a one-to-one basis, important though this is, but also to the availability of sufficient resources to ensure that care can be given competently, hence this is also a matter of public interest and should include concern over the quality of life of people on the receiving end of care as well as their unpaid carers. Care receiving is arguably the least well-developed aspect of the model. Tronto argued that responsiveness goes further than empathy. 'Rather than to put ourselves into their position … it suggests that we consider the other's position as that other expresses it' (Tronto 1993: 136). Tronto's characterisation of the '*we*' and the '*other*' in the care relationship is problematic as it portrays an individual with less agency and less power than the carer. Tronto (1993) argued that the 'phases' are to be considered as an integrated whole, which is inclusive of both givers and receivers of care. The model as a whole also recognises that an individual might be both giver and receiver of care, either simultaneously or at different times. It is unfortunate that the term 'phase' suggests a process or sequence, which tends to undermine the integrated nature of the model, which is one of its great strengths. For example, a failure to consider care from the perspective of the receiver is inherent in institutionalised services. Based on the integrated model developed by Fisher and Tronto (1991), it follows that in these circumstances, there is no ethic of care at all. Thus, the need is not to look for a way of correcting a part of the process but to rethink the entire basis on which the service has been established.

Tronto (2013) developed her model further to focus on the relationship between politics and care. To her four-phase model she added a fifth phase – *caring with*. She drew on Polanyi (2001 [1944]) whose critique of the late 19th- and early 20th-century market economy led him to the conclusion that there can never be a perfect market society because there will always be some members of the society who act against it, so creating a 'double movement' in which the principle of economic liberalism is in conflict with the principle of social protection. In Tronto's view, the growth of market forces under neoliberalism has been disastrous for democracy, ushering in an era of collective irresponsibility and inequity which has challenged the basis of democracy itself. Tronto (2017) identified three ways in which neoliberalism accounted for care: first as individual personal responsibility; second as a problem for the market; and third as a family matter. Attempts to rationalise and mechanise systems of care in line with market ideals are antithetical to caring, which demands time and resources and, as a result, she argued, these attempts have led to both a care deficit and a democracy deficit. In her conceptual model of '*caring with*', Tronto (2013) argued in favour establishing a democratic process to centre upon 'assigning responsibilities for care, and for ensuring that carers and those cared for are as capable as possible of participating in this assignment of responsibilities' (Tronto 2013: 7). The point of this process is not to try and equalise the burden of caring but to change the basis on which decisions are made about who should be responsible for care and in what ways. The starting point for this is the same as the starting point for the model developed earlier by Fisher and Tronto (1991): that people are not autonomous and independent individuals first, going on to form relationships, but vulnerable and interdependent first, achieving independence only because of having been cared for.

Tronto's is arguably the most well-developed of contemporary theories of care, but she has not ventured into drawing conclusions about the implications of her analysis for *policies*, having argued in 2013 that this is a job for those involved in democratic deliberations. Her analysis has been developed and critiqued by researchers from a wide range of disciplines, including policy studies (Sevenhuijsen 1998; Hankivsky 2005). In her critique of the Labour government's Third Way agenda, for example, Sevenhuijsen (2000) drew on the definition of care developed by Fisher and Tronto (1991) to argue that Third Way political agendas were focused too heavily on individualistic ideas of personal responsibility and strongly oriented towards an idealised view of the family. Tronto's critique of neoliberalism has also been taken up by political scientists and sociologists (see Lynch 2021, for example).

The ethics of care perspective, particularly in its earliest versions, has been subjected to critical commentary, much of which focused on the first generation of theorists for their tendency to equate care and gender. It is noteworthy that the ethics of care as a model is under constant development and criticism of its application should not be regarded as a reason for rejection of the model itself. Hankivsky (2014) argued that care ethicists had tended to 'tack on' issues of social diversity and inequality, rather than being conceptually inclusive, so that race and class are not treated in the same way as gender. She proposed that theoretical developments in intersectionality theory could assist in developing a care ethics that takes account of multiple social divisions and inequalities without privileging gender and that is more attuned to the exercise of power in the name of care. She noted, however, that the later work of care ethicists had been more attentive to socioeconomic and global inequalities (Hankivsky 2014).

Other critiques have focused on the tendency to conceptualise caring from the perspective of a caregiver and to overlook the perspective of the care receiver. Shakespeare (2006, 2013), for example, pointed out that the ethic of care does not engage adequately with the oppressive potential of care but tends to idealise the caring role, although he acknowledged that Sevenhuijsen (1998), Williams (2001) and others have recognised the potential for carers to be motivated not by an urge to protect but by an urge to meddle and control. For Shakespeare (2013), the advantages an ethic of care can bring to democratic citizenship and public discourse are undeniable, but he emphasises that it should also be recognised that an ethic of justice and equality is necessary in caring relationships. He commented on the need for all support and care systems to balance individualism and mutuality and to respect the needs and interests of both parties.

Herring (2014) was also critical of the lack of attention among feminist ethicists to the perspectives of those receiving care. As he argued, the social model of disability had identified disabling environments as causal factors in disability as opposed to the individual model that focused on health conditions and impairment, but he also pointed out that care was often part of this disabling environment because it individualised and problematised disability and emphasised the burdens of care. He concurred with the views of feminist ethicists, such as Tronto (1993), that the idea of autonomy and capacity claimed by traditional liberalism is misplaced, because we are all vulnerable and dependent on others for our physical and psychological wellbeing. To take these qualities as a given reality is relatively straightforward and in disability studies, he pointed out, there is a corresponding line of argument against the pressure on disabled people to maximise independence and fit in with 'normal' life. Herring was therefore critical of policies that emphasise the promotion of independence and the postponement of the need for care and support. But he went further than this, to argue that vulnerability and dependency should be *welcomed* as 'an aspect of many of the things people most value in their lives: relationships, intimacy, care' (Herring 2014: 14). He quoted Wiles (2011: 573), who said that vulnerability can be conceptualised not as fragility or weakness but as 'openness, susceptibility and receptiveness'. Herring (2014) also argued that it is by understanding human dependency and vulnerability that we can truly appreciate the importance of human rights.

As a feminist ethicist, Kittay (1999, 2011) has focused extensively on the meaning of dependency, based on her experience as the mother of a disabled daughter. For Kittay, physical dependency on others is our first experience of life as human beings and the entire life course is punctuated by periods of dependency. This acknowledgment of dependency enables a clearer understanding of the power imbalance that shapes care relationships. For some, a power imbalance between individuals in care relationships is problematic but Kittay differentiated between power (the ability of individuals to provide the necessary assistance) and domination (the abuse of trust in a care relationship). She argued that inequalities in power are quite compatible with justice and care unless the relationship becomes one of domination. Indeed, an ethic of care is needed because there is a power imbalance. Another of Kittay's distinctive contributions has been her perspective on 'nested dependencies'. She argued that care providers (unpaid carers) are also dependent on others, to prevent second-level vulnerabilities, such as poverty or ill health, that can befall them. These second-level vulnerabilities arise from the social conditions that shape care (or 'dependency work' as Kittay called it) and it is at this level that the need for a public ethic of care becomes clear because the role of supporting the one giving care must be a societal one. Kittay's contribution is valuable as a reminder that understanding dependency is essential to understanding care. Her perspective on 'nested dependencies' is a reminder of the interconnectedness of human beings, while her views on the power imbalance involved in care providing and receiving draw attention to the need for a public ethic of care to manage conflicts of interest and prevent domination and abuse.

These points are explored further in Chapter 6, with particular attention to their relevance to contemporary policies and practices.

What research tells us about unpaid care now

Research methods, approaches and organisation have changed significantly over the past three decades. One such development is the shift in perspective to embrace research 'with' rather than research 'on' carers and service users, which has, for example, generated research advisory panels as well as research teams that include 'experts by experience'. Partnerships between researchers and third-sector organisations have produced more detailed knowledge about the pressures on families with disabled children and adult members, incorporating the narrative accounts and experiences of carers and families into their findings. Indeed, such partnerships have increasingly become a condition of research funding. Research on unpaid care has also been incorporated into programmes and centres that facilitate cross-referencing between projects and place unpaid care into its wider social and policy context at national and international level. Unpaid care is now a vast field of study but remains disproportionately focused on the impact of unpaid care on carers – its cost to carers' health, financial status, social relationships and opportunities – than on relationships of care or the perspectives of people on the receiving end of care. Research on the impact of policies has been carried out by a number of researchers referred to in this book. Research units that have been active over the time period under discussion include, among others, those at the Social Policy Research Unit at the University of York; the London School of Economics Personal Social Services Research Unit; the School of Social Sciences at the University of Bangor; and the Sustainable Care Unit at the University of Sheffield.

Findings from a comprehensive scoping review of carer-related research and knowledge produced by Henwood et al (2019) were organised – conveniently for the purposes of this discussion – into four main parts: carer variables; type of care; the impact of care; and support and carers (see also Larkin et al 2019). They offered an analysis of each part. The 'carer variables' part focused on the nature of relationships (spouse, child, adult child) as well as gender, age and ethnicity. They observed that research that focuses on one part of a caring dyad misses out on the complexity of a caring relationship and on the potential of caring networks. Henwood et al (2019) also identified a growth of research on 'hidden carers': those that do not identify themselves as carers per se for various reasons, or who might be in a subset that is harder to identify and locate, such as lesbian, gay, bisexual and trans (LGBTQI) or minority ethnic carers. Research on the type of care, the second grouping, highlighted the diversity of caring. The frequency of types identified were, in descending order, older people, dementia, mental health, end of life, cancer and long-term health conditions, although these types often overlapped. Areas of tension related to identity and autonomy were also identified, the example given being mental health, where the need for care fluctuates, meaning that a relative does not meet the common view of a carer as one who provides regular and substantial care. Other areas of tension identified were conflicts between carer and the person they support, as well as ethical problems in relation to the custodial nature of care, such as the use of telemonitoring. The impact of caring upon carers was the single largest category of all the analyses reviewed by Henwood et al (2019), amounting to almost 40 per cent of all themes identified. They concluded that the complexity of carers' responses to the 'burden' of caring underlines the importance of not making assumptions about the burdensomeness of care simply by reference to the health condition of the person supported. Research suggested that carers' coping strategies were often linked to the need for information and dealing with uncertainty. The impact of caring on carers' health was the most frequently identified theme, not straightforwardly evident or causal and often mixed with the health of the person cared for. As Henwood et al (2019) commented, this is an indication of the difficulties of distinguishing between objective and subjective dimensions as well as causes and consequences of health and care. The impact of caring on carers' employment was another theme, which had particular implications for social care policies, given the relationship between alternative forms of care and carers' ability to participate in paid employment. The final grouping – support and carers – focused on difficulties for carers within the care system, including in the assessment of needs, evidence on respite, which has been equivocal, and examples of interventions, such as professionally led support groups and psychosocial support for carers of people with dementia.

The key messages that Henwood et al (2019) drew from their review include the diversity of research and knowledge, the diversity of caring situations researched, the importance of a perspective on the complexity of care relationships, and the gaps in knowledge related to specific groups, including minority Black and ethnic and LGBTQI carers. The diverse needs of different types of carers, including those arising at different points of the life course, are also a focus of interest. Another point of interest raised is the need for more longitudinal data that would enhance understanding of the process of caring relationships over time. Given this extensive diversity, it is not surprising that they also concluded that when it comes to support for unpaid care, this should be tailored rather than one-size-fits-all.

Many of the themes raised by Henwood et al (2019) point to the way in which carers have become conceptually separated from those they care for, even though the evidence suggests that their needs and interests are deeply entwined with those of the individuals they care for. They also reiterated the points made by Nolan et al (1996) discussed earlier, that over-reliance on cross-sectional design in research has resulted in an inadequate level of understanding of the dynamic nature of care relationships over time and that researchers have been disproportionately interested in the impact of the caring role on carers. As Milne and Larkin (2015) and Larkin et al (2019) pointed out, findings from this 'gathering and evaluating' approach to research has amassed a great deal of detail and reinforced this dominant view of the negative impacts of caring. Moreover, research of this type has produced fragmented and uneven results because of specific fields of interest, such as unpaid care of people with dementia. On the other hand, studies that they referred to as 'conceptualising and theorising' about care, including the work of feminist ethicists and disability theorists, took a broader view of care, examining the carer identity, the gendered nature of care and professional perceptions of the carer role. Henwood et al (2019) called for a shift in thinking about research on unpaid care, to locate care within a continuum of ordinary relationships rather than a dichotomy of carer and cared for, and to engage with the complexity of care so that a better understanding about care and carers can underpin policies. Attempting to identify the influence of research findings on policies can be a dismal experience when evidence is produced repeatedly to apparently little effect. As Larkin et al (2019) pointed out, research of the gathering and evaluating type has not had a positive effect on practice while research of the conceptualising and theorising type is barely visible in the discourse surrounding policy making.

The discussion in this book looks also at the reverse process – the ways in which policies influence knowledge about care. The capacity of the policy agenda to shape ideas about care has been a significant development since 1990 and has extended to researchers in terms of how their research questions are formulated and how decisions about research funding are made. The place of unpaid care within the social care system has become normalised as a resource for local authorities to draw upon. It is unsurprising, therefore, that researchers often focus on specific types of care relationships, or specific needs, and seek answers to questions about the efficacy of interventions without questioning underpinning assumptions about the normalised exploitation of unpaid care. When placed in an historical context, the long-term trends in research provoke questions, such as why has there been increasing research attention to carers' resilience and capacity to cope over the past three decades? Why is there increasing research interest in enabling carers in paid employment to manage the stresses of their situation, when their statutory rights are still so limited? This is not to denigrate the efforts of researchers – that would be hypocritical – but to point to the importance of seeing the bigger picture beyond the world of professional practice and existing policy trends.

Conclusion

Several themes in research have endured over three decades. For example, Parker (1994) called for researchers to pay more attention to caring

Table 3.1: Outline of policies to support unpaid carers in the UK

	England	Scotland	Wales	Northern Ireland
1995	Carers (Recognition and Services) Act	Carers (Recognition and Services) Act	Carers (Recognition and Services) Act	
1999	*Caring for Carers* Strategy	Scottish Strategy for Carers		
2000	Carers and Disabled Children Act		*Caring about Carers*: Carers Strategy in Wales Implementation Plan	
			Carers and Disabled Children Act	
2002		Community Care and Health (Scotland) Act		Carers and Direct Payments (Northern Ireland) Act
2004	Carers (Equal Opportunities) Act		Carers (Equal Opportunities) Act	
2006				*Caring for Carers*: Carers Strategy for Northern Ireland
2006	Work and Families Act			
2007	Pensions Act			
2008	Strategy: *Carers at the Heart of 21st Century Families and Communities*			
2009				Review of the support provision for carers
2010	*Recognised, Valued and Supported: Next Steps for the Carers Strategy*	Caring Together: The Carers Strategy for Scotland 2010–2015	Carers Strategies (Wales) Measure	
2010	Equality Act			
2013		Social Care (Self-Directed Support) Act		
2014	Care Act		Social Services and Wellbeing (Wales) Act	
	Children and Families Act			
2016		Carers (Scotland) Act		Expert Advisory Panel on Adult Care and Support

(continued)

Table 3.1: Outline of policies to support unpaid carers in the UK (continued)

	England	Scotland	Wales	Northern Ireland
2018	Carers Action Plan 2018–2020	Carers Charter		
2021		Carers (Scotland) Act 2016: Implementation Plan 2021–2023	*Strategy for Unpaid Carers*, Wales	
2022	Health and Care Act		Charter for Unpaid Carers	Reform of Adult Social Care consultation paper

twin aims of his Bill were to give carers the right to a separate assessment of their needs and to empower local authorities to provide services that would support them. The Bill expanded the definition of 'private carers' in the NHSCC Act, 1990 to include children and young people as well as the parents of disabled children. It was calculated then that this would include around 1.5 million carers.

> [A] 'private carer' means a person (not being a person employed to provide the care in question by any body in the exercise of its functions under any enactment) who is providing care on a regular basis to a disabled person (including a disabled person who is a minor) and includes such persons who are the children (including minors), parents, spouses or other relations of the disabled person for whom they care. (House of Commons 1994)

Carers were therefore defined not by age nor by their relationship to the person they cared for. What qualified them for an assessment of need was given in Section 1(1) of the Carers (Recognition and Services) Act 1995, as follows: 'An individual who provides or intends to provide a substantial amount of care on a regular basis for another person' (DH 1995). The Carers (Recognition and Services) Act, 1995 applied with a few variations throughout the UK and was the first piece of legislation to recognise, albeit to a limited extent, the needs of carers as separate from the needs of those they supported. Where an individual was being assessed for community care services, and where that person's carer requested it, the local authority was required to carry out a separate assessment of the carer's needs for services. Their entitlement to separate attention was therefore stronger than had been the case under the community care legislation but not broad enough to cover all carers as it was restricted to those caring for an individual already in the care system. Indeed, when the Bill was presented to the House of Lords, Lord Carter explained that the Bill did not seek to separate the needs of the carers and those they cared for but to promote a holistic approach which would avoid the possibility of two assessment procedures running in parallel.

There were different perceptions in the Bill of what recognition entailed. For example, explaining its basic philosophy, Lord Carter stated that 'it is crucial to ensure that local authorities take proper account of carers' circumstances when carrying out an assessment of need for community care services of the person being cared for' (Hansard 1995). At the same time, Baroness Seear, President of the Carers National Association at the time, commented that the Bill 'shows that the carer's position is at last ... understood for what it is. The carer is not just an appendage of the person who needs to be looked after'. Thus, while both emphasise the importance of recognition, for one that involves taking into consideration the carer in relation to the person they support while for the other it involves acknowledging a separate identity with specific separate needs.

The services available to carers were envisaged as those that would enable the carer to continue caring, reflecting an instrumental approach to support. Local authorities were empowered – but not required – to meet carers' needs, which meant that if it appeared that carers could continue without support then there was no obligation on the part of local authorities to offer them any support at all. Having conducted an assessment, the local authority would decide whether the assessed needs called for the provision of services and, if so, these were recorded as 'eligible needs' that must be met. During the process of debating the Bill, flexibility and choice were emphasised and local authorities urged not to limit their services to personal care but offer practical help in the home where needed.

Respite – or having a break from caring – also featured as an important demand of carers and there was increasing awareness that greater variation was needed in the type of arrangements offered, beyond temporary accommodation in care homes. The Disabled Persons and Carers (Short Term Breaks) Bill, 1996 introduced by Lord Rix, a prominent supporter of Mencap, picked up on this point, arguing for more personalised approaches to breaks (Hansard 1996). In 1998, following the election of the Labour government, the Bill was reintroduced in the House of Commons by Huw Edwards MP (Hansard 1998). The aim of the Bill was to make respite care universally available to carers, to raise the standard of respite care and to increase the variety of services. Although this Bill did not complete its passage, several of its aims were incorporated into the Carers and Disabled Children Act, 2000, discussed later in this chapter in the section 'Modernising social care'.

Implementation of the Carers (Recognition and Services) Act, 1995 was a challenge for local authorities, which already faced the additional costs involved in the implementation of the NHSCC Act, 1990 at a time of reduced resources (Holzhausen and Jackson 1997b). Some were reluctant to take on additional areas of responsibility and to conduct assessments when there were inadequate services to respond to assessed need. In practice, the terminology of the legislation, intended to be broad and inclusive, proved challenging. What did 'substantial' and 'regular' mean? How would differences in carers' levels of health and fitness apply? Should an 80-year-old and a 40-year-old be doing the same amount of care to qualify for an assessment? On this point, the Policy Guidance simply advised that the terms substantial and regular 'should be interpreted in their everyday sense' (DH 1996: 10). There was also a lack of consistency over the meaning of the term 'eligibility' and local authorities were expected to publish their own definitions, introducing another element of inequality between them. Although the 1995 Act was a significant breakthrough for carers, especially in relation to recognition, it did not meet their demands for support services (Holzhausen and Jackson 1997a). The Policy Guidance on the Act warned that the impact of the Act would be gradual and urged local authorities to inform carers of their entitlements so that progress could be made.

The Labour government: strategies on unpaid care in the context of devolution and modernisation

After the general election of 1997, the incoming Labour government maintained the tight financial constraints of the outgoing Conservative administration, while pursuing their 'Third Way' political and economic strategy, which sought to demonstrate that social justice and economic efficiency were not mutually opposed. Modernisation of the public sector was a key element of the Third Way, which included the modernisation of local authority social services (or social care, as it came to be described). Although the policy rhetoric was against the privatisation of services, the reality was that the mixed economy of welfare became more firmly established under Labour.

Devolution was a priority of the government's agenda and the year 1998 saw the formation of the Scottish Parliament and the National Assemblies for Wales and Northern Ireland. The four populations differed in several respects, which had implications for both demand for and provision of health and social care services. First, there were differences in levels of need: for example, the average age and levels of disability of the population in Wales were then (and remain) higher than in the other three countries. Second, there were differences in the cost of provision: Scotland is more sparsely populated with consequently higher costs in provision (Atkins et al 2021). Third, there were differences in the pre-existing organisation of services: in Northern Ireland, the integrated system of health and social care already offered free nursing care at home. There were also differences in the powers available to the devolved administrations. In contrast to the Scottish Parliament, neither the Welsh nor the Northern Ireland Assemblies had powers to enact primary legislation. In the subsequent years, devolution proved to be a 'dynamic and contested process' (Mooney et al 2006) and policy priorities differed in certain respects. For example, there was greater political commitment in Scotland and Wales than in England to collaborative approaches to health and social care provision and less interest in a marketised system (Andrews and Martin 2010; Atkins et al 2021). In both Scotland and Wales, prescription charges for medication were abolished and in 2002 the Scottish government introduced free social care to individuals over 65. At the time of writing, all three devolved governments spend more per head of population on care than is spent in England. There are similarities in policy priorities, including enabling individuals to live in their own homes; greater individual choice for service users and carers; and more 'personalised' services as well as support for unpaid carers. After 2008, austerity policies introduced by the Westminster government resulted in stringent budget cuts which applied throughout the UK, affecting the financial settlements made between Westminster and the devolved governments. Consequently, spending on social care has never kept up with demand and local authorities in all four countries have struggled to meet their statutory obligations. In addition, in Northern Ireland, the long period of conflict and direct rule from Westminster from 1972 to 1999 left health and social care services with limited opportunities to develop innovative policies in health or social care (Ham et al 2013).

National strategies for carers

Following devolution, strategies to develop support for unpaid carers were introduced at an early stage in all four countries: in 1999 in England and Scotland, in 2000 in Wales and 2002 in Northern Ireland (see Table 3.1). All four strategies emphasised partnerships between statutory departments, acknowledging the importance of carers' needs beyond health and social care services, and all paid attention to carers in paid employment and young carers in education. In addition, all strategies acknowledged the diversity of carers and committed the governments to more personalised forms of services to reflect this diversity. All strategies encouraged the involvement of carers as 'stakeholders' in local service planning and development. In many ways, the carers strategies reflected Third Way thinking, since they were an attempt to conjoin principles of justice and social inclusion on the one hand with economic efficiency on the other. Supporting carers was presented as an ideal way of keeping down the cost of social care, providing those who needed care with the opportunity to remain in their own homes, and promoting recognition and a better quality of life for carers. In addition, support for carers was presented as *morally* desirable because of carers' value to society at large. Recognition of carers was crucially important, not only because of their essential role and function in caring but also because they exemplify good citizenship. Carers' involvement as stakeholders in policy making is also a mark of recognition of their citizen status. In the Westminster Parliament, the Scottish Parliament and Welsh Senedd (as the Welsh Assembly became) specialist, all-party interest groups on carers continue to play an important role in informing politicians and influencing policies, acting as the authentic voice of carers. The Carers National Association (itself the product of an earlier merger in 1988) renamed itself Carers UK in 2001 in order to better reflect its position as a member organisation (Cook 2007). It now enjoys a position as a key source of evidence and information for policy makers.

The first national strategy for carers, introduced in England in 1999, *Caring about Carers: A National Strategy for Carers*, was described as a 'new, substantial policy package' based on a partnership between central and local governments, the NHS and private and voluntary organisations. Its stated aim was to give carers more control over the range, nature and timing of services as well as the amount of care they provide, their participation in employment, education and their communities. According to Paul Boateng, the Minister of Health at the time, it gave carers a voice at the heart of government (HM Government 1999a). Information, support and care were key areas of focus. *Information* was related to the need for a better understanding *about* carers and it was in this document that the intention to include a question on caring in the 2001 Census was announced publicly. Information was also *for* carers, related to what they should know about services and the cost of these, as well as about the health conditions and care needs of the individuals they supported. *Support* for carers focused on local health and social services as well as housing adaptations and the use of technology in the home. Health professionals, including general practitioners (GPs), were encouraged to embrace carers' health as part of their role in prevention and health promotion. *Care* for carers referred to community-based services, including, importantly, the provision of regular breaks from caring. For the first time, local authorities in England were provided with a ring-fenced fund to pay for breaks for carers and guidance given to local authorities set out standards of good practice.

The English strategy advanced the agenda of providing services for carers *in their own right*. It dispensed with the condition that the person being supported must have a needs assessment for their carer to qualify for one, as this was perceived as undervaluing the role of carers. Another perceptible change was the view that 'helping carers is one of the best ways of helping the people they care for' (HM Government 1999a: 12), which reinforced a shift in thinking about carers as a focus of services rather than merely featuring in care packages of the individuals they cared for. To this end, regular breaks for carers were presented as a means of empowering them. There were also reforms to existing cash benefits, which applied to all parts of the UK. A new benefit, the Carer's Allowance, was introduced for individuals that provided at least 35 hours a week to a person who received a qualifying disability benefit. The Allowance was paid to one carer supporting one person. Enabling carers to take up paid employment was also a priority in the English strategy, which reflected the Labour government's emphasis on paid work as a route to social inclusion, citizenship and opportunity.

Following the establishment of the parliament in Holyrood, the Scottish government embarked on its own community care system and introduced its national carers strategy, in 1999 (Scottish Government 1999). This included many of the same themes as the English strategy, particularly the emphasis on flexibility in service provision, more personalised services and the provision of resources to cover the cost of regular breaks from caring. It also focused on young carers who were portrayed as particularly disadvantaged because of the impact of caring on their life chances. Its four priorities were respite, standards, legislation and information. As was the case in England, there had been widespread consultation with carers, which had highlighted carers' demands for better quality respite services.

The Scottish strategy also promoted the rights of carers to information about their entitlements (including their entitlement to assessments as well as to pensions). As in the English strategy, improved information about carers was a key aim and the Scottish Census of 2001 was earmarked as a means of achieving this. Service providers were urged to reach out to 'hidden' carers to ensure that people caring for relatives would have the information they needed to come forward for help. The Scottish strategy placed a heavy emphasis on separating the rights of carers from the rights of the people they supported and on promoting services to carers 'in their own right'. It also enhanced the status and influence of carers' organisations as active participants in the development of health and social care services as well as the training of GPs, primary care teams and social workers. When the strategy was introduced to the Scottish Parliament in 1999, it was given the stamp of approval from carers' organisations (Scottish Parliament 1999).

Caring about Carers: The Carers Strategy in Wales, Implementation Plan (Welsh Assembly Government 2000) was described as a first practical step towards addressing the needs of carers, indicating that for the administration in Wales, support for carers was to be an ongoing policy concern. Indeed, the plan committed the National Assembly for Wales to annual reviews of the strategy and a Carers Strategy Review Panel was established with a view to ensuring effective implementation. The Implementation Plan in Wales highlighted similar priorities to those in England and Scotland: information for and about carers; health and social care services for carers; support for young carers; and support for carers in employment. Giving carers greater control over the range, nature and timing of services was a key element of the Implementation Plan, which was intended to promote carers' rights and cater for the diversity of caregiving settings (Seddon et al 2010). One measure introduced specifically in Wales was the provision of six weeks' free home care on discharge from hospital. The strategy was evaluated in conjunction with developments in other services, including mental health, the NHS and social services for older and disabled people, in line with the community-based approach to service provision developing in Wales.

Influenced by the other strategies already produced in England, Scotland and Wales, the Northern Ireland Assembly's 2002 Carers Strategy emphasised five main principles: partnerships between services and unpaid carers; the personalisation of services for individual carers; the right of carers to have 'a life outside of caring', including through paid employment and education; the freedom of individuals to choose whether or not to become carers without professionals making assumptions about their choice; and the requirement that government should invest in carers through providing practical support, such as information and training for carers to enhance their ability to fulfil their roles (DHSSPS 2002). The theme of partnership between professionals and unpaid carers was reflected in all four strategies, albeit in differing ways. The Northern Ireland integrated Health and Social Services Boards embodied partnerships that differed from other parts of the UK, although not all commentators were convinced that integration between health and social services was as successful on the ground as it was on paper (Hudson and Henwood 2002).

Modernising social care

The Labour government's modernisation agenda, applied across the public sector, aimed to improve efficiency and obtain better value for money. The Audit Commission, set up in 1983 to inspect local authorities' economy, efficiency and effectiveness in service provision, was expanded to include a role in examining local authorities' approaches to service improvements. In social care an additional aim was to promote the rights of citizens, through consultative activities (Humphrey 2003). The turn of the 21st century saw a high level of activity in policies on health and social care in England. A series of National Service Frameworks (NSFs) were developed in the NHS in England to initiate improvements in the quality of services. Each of these Frameworks referred to unpaid carers. In the NSF on Mental Health (DH 1999b), for example, it was pointed out that without better attention to the needs of carers it would be impossible to achieve the quality standards set in the Framework. It stated that carers of people with mental health problems on a Care Programme Approach (especially those caring for people with serious mental health problems and dementia) should have a separate assessment of their needs repeated on at least an annual basis and have their own written care plan, implemented in discussion with them (Arksey et al 2002). The NSF on Older People was advised by a Carers' Focus Group and, although progress on this NSF was stalled by subsequent reorganisations in the NHS, the practice of including carers' groups and organisations in the policy process was maintained, while the 1999 Health Act referred to unpaid carers as 'partners' (Hirst 2001). Together, these developments demonstrate a growing awareness of carers on the part of service planners and managers and of the effectiveness of carers' campaigns, which gained them an officially sanctioned place in service planning at the local level. At the same time, the Labour government came in for criticism for its centralised controls over local service provision, especially as its policy agenda contained inconsistencies. For example, the NSFs had set out how things should be done to ensure local level service planning reflected national (English) priorities, but local authorities were also being urged to consult local citizens, including carers, about their views on local service priorities.

The Carers and Disabled Children Act, 2000 (which applied in England and Wales) codified in law the aims of the English strategy for carers in several ways. It gave carers the right to an assessment of their needs, independent of any assessment of the person they were supporting and enabled local authorities to provide services directly to carers. Carers were given the right to ask for an assessment, but it was also expected that if a local authority employee was assessing the needs of a service user, they should inform that person's carer that they also were entitled to an assessment. Assessments determined whether an individual carer was eligible for services, how their health and wellbeing could be maintained and the best ways of meeting their needs. The scope of what constituted appropriate support was broadened. Cash in lieu of services in the form of direct payments was encouraged and vouchers were introduced to give carers greater choice and control over where and how they took a break from caring. Parallel arrangements were made for carers in the 16–17 age group, through amendments to the Children Act, 1989. Services for adult carers included advice and information as well as 'sign posting' to carers' support groups or carers' centres. Improved choice was an underlying theme of the legislation, and the pressure was on local authorities to be flexible and innovative in their support arrangements. The introduction of direct payments and vouchers promoted not only flexibility and choice but also self-management, self-help and independence as key principles of social care. The view that carers and service users were the experts in understanding their own needs had gained ground by 2000. In this spirit, the Practice Guidance that accompanied the Carers and Disabled Children

Act, 2000, urged practitioners to focus on *carer-defined outcomes* to overcome the tendency to think in terms of support based on existing services (DH 2001a). As Seddon et al (2007) pointed out, what was meant by a 'positive outcome' was not entirely clear but one potential outcome identified was the carer's ability to take up or continue paid employment. Support for carers was therefore not necessarily linked directly to their caring role but was intended to make it easier and more convenient for them to fit their caring responsibilities into their lives more generally.

Support for carers was also integrated into the 2001 Strategy for Learning Disability – Valuing People (DH 2001b). This expanded on some of the themes already covered. For example, in developing knowledge about carers, local authorities were urged to find out about the numbers of parents (especially those aged 70 and over) who were carers of adult sons and daughters with learning disabilities and to develop care plans for the future of those sons and daughters. Also in 2003, the Westminster government passed the Community Care (Delayed Discharges) Act, which required social services departments to determine what support would be provided for an individual carer when the person they supported was ready to be discharged from hospital. This Act was applicable in both England and Wales, although subsequently the government in Wales developed its own strategy. In Scotland, the Delayed Discharges Action Plan, passed in 2002, reflected Scotland's more collectivist approach to social care. Delayed discharges in England and Wales incurred fines on local authorities while in Scotland there were no fines but a requirement on both health and social care services to develop joint agreements (Godfrey and Townsend 2009).

The Community Care and Health (Scotland) Act, 2002 introduced free personal care for older people living either in their own homes or in care homes and created new rights for carers, who would be supported through social care services. Personal care was defined as 'help with personal hygiene, continence management, assistance with eating and mobility, counselling and support services, assistance with medication and simple treatments and personal assistance such as help getting up and going to bed' (Bowes and Bell 2007: 436). In 2018 the right to free personal care was extended to disabled people under the age of 65, when the European Court of Justice ruled in favour of Amanda Kopel, the wife of Frank Kopel, who was diagnosed with dementia at the age of 59. She had claimed that her husband was being unfairly treated on the grounds of his age.

The Guidance on Sections 8–12 of this Act, which were of greatest direct relevance to carers, supplanted the guidance issued under the Carers (Recognition and Services) Act, 1995 and marked Scotland's divergence from what had been the UK-wide approach to support for carers. A key point of divergence was the identification of unpaid carers as partners in providing care with paid professionals and care workers. This was described as a crucially important underpinning principle influencing all help and advice given to carers. Thus, the Community Care and Health Scotland Act, 2002 did not seek to develop services for carers but to provide the *resources* necessary for them to carry out their function. The carer's 'ability to care' was a key term used in relation to a carer's assessment, to determine if a carer was capable and willing to care and what would make their role sustainable. At the same time, Scotland's approach to social care was already developing a more integrated approach, with 'single shared assessments' of carers being the preferred method. No one professional group had responsibility for carers' assessments but it was decided that staff in health, social care or the voluntary sector should be involved, calling on the expertise of others as needed. Like the legislation in England, the provision of respite or short breaks was regarded as a high priority. This was consistent with their perception of carers as co-providers of care who were entitled to a regular break to enable them to continue in their role.

The overall policy emphasis in Wales at this time was not on the Westminster government's modernisation agenda but on developing a uniquely Welsh approach to a community-based model of service provision, which included an enhanced role for the voluntary sector. In relation to carers, the voluntary sector was regarded as important not only as a means of identifying and supporting individual carers but also as a way of promoting carers' influence through their organisations and networks including their representation on the Carers Strategy Review Panel. Responding to the diversity of the carer population, a good practice guide on working with minority Black and ethnic carers was published: *Challenging the Myth 'They Look After Their Own'* (Welsh Government/Llywodraeth Cymru 2003). Support for carers in paid employment was embedded in the European 'EQUAL' initiative that sought ways of improving equality of opportunity in employment. In relation to carers, this pre-Brexit policy provided for European funds to be used in Wales, to facilitate carers' access to employment and developing more carer-friendly conditions of employment.

The Carers and Direct Payments (Northern Ireland) Act, 2002 required the Health and Social Services Trusts to inform carers of their right to have an assessment of needs, irrespective of the decision of the person they support to accept or refuse an assessment. The purpose of an assessment under this legislation was to determine a carer's eligibility for support, to identify the needs of the carer and to see if those needs can be met (DHSSPS 2002). Guidance on this legislation was updated in 2005 to include additional guidance concerning a 'carer-centred' approach to assessment and the use of a single comprehensive assessment tool (Taylor 2012). This was originally designed with older service users in mind but was being further developed for other groups, including carers. In the same year, *Valuing Carers: A Strategy for Carers in Northern Ireland* was published (DHSSPS 2002). This listed 19 recommendations, with four main areas of action identified – information and training, support services, employment and help for young carers. Following the recommendations of the report, unpaid carers were included as a priority group in the Northern Ireland Executive's Promoting Social Inclusion Programme and an interdepartmental Carers Working Group was also established by the Executive.

Developing the carers' rights agenda

The rights of carers in England and Wales were consolidated further through the Carers (Equal Opportunities) Act, 2004. Three changes to the law were introduced. First, local authorities were required to inform individuals identified as carers that they might be entitled to an assessment under the 1995 and 2000 Acts. Second, local authorities were required to take into consideration whether the carer works or undertakes any form of education, training or leisure activity during the process of an assessment. Third, the Act promoted co-operation between local authorities and other authorities in relation to services for carers. Like the Carers (Recognition and Services) Act, 1995 and the Carers and Disabled Children Act, 2000 before it, the Carers (Equal Opportunities) Act, 2004 was introduced to parliament through a Private Members' Bill. Hywel Francis MP, the sponsor, argued that:

> The Bill's provisions are relatively modest. They will improve information for carers about their rights and will enhance the choices open to them through work, education and leisure. For individuals, the personal impact of the Bill could be huge. It aims to change the culture to acknowledge that carers have a right to information so that they can make choices about their lives, and a right to 'have a life', as one carer put it, beyond their caring responsibilities. (Hansard 2004)

Clements et al (2011) argued that the Carers (Equal Opportunities) Act, 2004, marked a shift in approach from the previously dominant focus on sustaining the caring role to a new focus on tackling social exclusion among carers and enabling them to have a life beyond caring. The Act could therefore be regarded as a further step in decoupling the rights of unpaid carers from the rights of the people they cared for. Another development was the requirement on local authorities to develop partnership arrangements with local voluntary and independent organisations, employers and health service providers to promote the wellbeing of carers as a shared endeavour. Supporting carers' opportunities to take up paid employment was a key element of the Act and was very much in line with the Labour government's wider promotion of paid work in place of cash benefits. Local authorities were urged to consider a carer's wish to continue or take up paid employment or to embark on training and education when carrying out a service user's assessment of needs. At the same time, employers were urged to make provision for their employees who were also unpaid carers, by offering greater flexibility in their hours of work and consideration for time off when they needed to attend medical or other appointments with the person they cared for.

A report by Care 21 (2006) on *The Future of Unpaid Care in Scotland* recommended a rights-based approach, including carers' rights to choose to care or not as well as to flexible employment, financial support information, practical support, regular breaks adequate housing, training transport, recreational and educational opportunities. The report argued that an unpaid carer's rights should be equalised with those of disabled people and paid staff. An example of the need for this action was that while health and safety legislation upheld the right of employed care staff not to carry out a care function perceived to be risky, the same protection was not extended to unpaid carers.

The Equality Act, 2010

Despite the additional rights given to carers across the UK under the 2006 Work and Families Act, carers continued to experience discrimination at work. The 2010 Equality Act was intended to address their concerns through the concept of associative discrimination, incorporating into law the decision of the 2008 European Court of Justice decision in the case of Sharon Coleman, the mother of a disabled child. Ms Coleman had claimed that she had been unfairly dismissed as she had been treated less favourably than parents of non-disabled children. The decision of the court was that the concept of direct discrimination and harassment extended to employees who are associated with disabled people, although not themselves disabled. Clements et al (2011) noted that when the Carers (Equal Opportunities) Act, 2004 was going through its parliamentary procedures, Hywel Francis MP had proposed an amendment to the Disability Discrimination Act, 1995, along these lines to make it unlawful to discriminate against carers as people 'associated with disabled people'. The 2008 decision in the European Court of Justice finally brought this about. The Equality Act, 2010 also imposed duties on the public sector in its provisions for disabled people, which were intended to compel public bodies to consider the impact of any new policy initiative on carers. Clements et al (2011) regarded this as part of the cultural shift towards regarding carers in their own right rather than as unpaid service providers. The introduction of associative discrimination and the public sector equality duty was significant in terms of policy on unpaid care and it galvanised campaigns for unpaid carers' rights. At the time of writing, Carers UK is conducting a campaign to have unpaid caring recognised as the Tenth Protected Characteristic under the Equality Act, 2010, to improve on their position and to achieve a level playing field with the nine groups currently protected. This would, for example, generate a duty to make reasonable adjustments for unpaid carers in employment.

Putting People First

Under the Community Care (Direct Payments) Act, 1996, local authorities in England had been given the power to provide cash in lieu of services. In the UK as in other countries disabled people's demands for greater choice and control over the support they received were increasing. For many, the provision of cash was an important step towards achieving their civil rights as adults. In the Carers and Disabled Children Act, 2000, direct payments or vouchers had been made available for parents of disabled children and disabled adults, but it was after 2007 that this policy came into its own, as a core element of public services under the Labour government's modernisation agenda (Needham and Glasby 2014). The Concordat 'Putting People First' aimed to transform the system of social care. To this end, partnerships between local authority social care services and independent providers were promoted and local authority management became increasingly corporate in nature, with oversight of budgets to be spent in the voluntary and commercial sectors.

Personal budgets and direct payments were secured as the generally accepted way of working with all service users (DH 2007) rather than as an option for a minority. Personal budgets, influenced by the work carried out in Scotland by the social enterprise 'In Control' (Needham and Glasby 2014), was a method of attaching a monetary value to interventions in response to individuals' assessed needs. A crucial aspect of this was that the individual service user should be involved in decisions about how the money should be spent. This required greater openness and transparency about how much was being spent and in what way, although care managers maintained overall control over the expenditure. Direct payments were a result of campaigns by disabled people for cash in lieu of services to give them greater control over expenditure. Direct payments often involved the employment of a personal assistant, either directly or through an agency operating on behalf of the disabled person. Family members could be employed as personal assistants as long as they were not living in the same household. The amount of money allocated to individuals either in their personal budget or direct payment was determined through a new Resource Allocation System, which went hand in hand with proposed self-assessment of needs. A programme of evaluation of the Individual Budgets pilot project – the IBSEN study – was set up in 2005 (Glendinning et al 2008) but before it reported the government in England pressed ahead with the implementation of the personalisation agenda, albeit with some modifications. One such was a change in the rights of people with learning disabilities to obtain a direct payment. There had been moves in some local authorities to provide support services to enable people to obtain direct payments, irrespective of their capacity to make decisions. In 2009 the Department of Health issued guidance to legalise this practice and to introduce the role of 'suitable person' as the payee and manager of the direct payment. Hence, many parents or close relatives of children and adults with learning disabilities became 'suitable persons' in law (Coles 2015). In Wales there was a more cautious approach, with a slower rollout of the policy to allow for the results of an evaluation but personalisation in the form of 'citizen directed support' became part of its strategy for social services in 2011.

By 2010, as only 4 per cent of carers had received an assessment of need, the choice between receiving a direct payment or services was an irrelevance (Mitchell et al 2014). In addition, it was becoming evident that policies to support carers were sometimes at odds with those promoting personalisation. Clements et al (2008), for example, pointed to concerns over the way the personalisation programme in practice had become 'delinked' from the statutory framework of care in the community – a framework that included the legislation to support carers. As the personalisation agenda became embedded in local authority practices, it became increasingly clear that carers were often overlooked in decisions about granting direct payments. The IBSEN study, for example, found that very few of the local authorities they reviewed had offered carers a self-assessment form, without which carers' entitlement to a direct payment could not be established (Mitchell et al 2014). There were also differences between service user groups, with working-aged disabled people and individuals with sensory impairments more likely than older people, learning disabled people or individuals with mental health issues to be offered a direct payment. Early evaluations of the personalisation agenda suggested that unpaid carers had a large amount of additional work to do, supporting the service user in managing their budget, which could include administrative assistance and help with the employment of paid personal assistants. Clements et al (2008) noted that many of the case examples that were cited at the time to highlight the positive aspects of direct payments were successful precisely *because* unpaid carers had contributed significant amounts of time and energy into making them work. Nevertheless, there was also evidence that despite the additional work involved, many carers appreciated having greater choice and control (Mitchell et al 2014). Another important point raised at the time by Clements et al (2008) was that the new Resources Allocation System, the formula through which the financial value of an individual budget was calculated, assumed that individuals living with a carer were entitled to half the amount of financial support than those who were not. This, they argued, raised serious questions about carers' basic human rights.

New strategies for carers

The new Carers Strategy for England – *Carers at the Heart of 21st Century Families and Communities: 'A Caring System on Your Side. A Life of Your Own'* – was introduced in 2008 as a ten-year programme. It emphasised the widespread nature of caring, that caring is a 'part of our lives' (HM Government 2008: 5) and that it should be made easier for carers to fit in their caring responsibilities around the rest of their lives. A caring system 'on your side' was thus intended to give carers the sense that they are supported, for example, through the provision of personalised, tailor-made services, financial support and regular breaks. The NHS was also identified as essential to this strategy, the aim being to provide regular health checks for carers and better awareness on the part of GPs and other health professionals about the distinct needs of carers. This Strategy was also linked to the wider policy, expressed in Putting People First, of developing more personalised services and transforming social care, but it also signalled expectations about unpaid care. Thus, while the promotion of independence and choice were key to the development of personalisation, the additional calls on unpaid carers were identified. The Strategy referred to the 'sacrifices that so many of us are prepared to make' (HM Government 2008: 2) to continue the process of deinstitutionalisation. There was great disappointment among carers that the Strategy did not announce an increase in the Carer's Allowance. Instead, a benefits review was set up, which, as was said at the time, did nothing to address the immediate problem of financial hardship among carers.

The strategy was updated in 2010 when the newly elected Conservative and Liberal Democrat Coalition government linked support for carers to their wider agenda of the 'Big Society'. The updated version focused on prioritising four areas of activity, based on consultations with the Standing Commission on Carers: support for early self-identification as a carer; enabling those with caring responsibilities to fulfil their potential in employment and education; personalised support for both carers and those they support; and supporting carers to remain mentally and physically well.

In 2010 the *Carers Strategy for Scotland 2010–2015* (Scottish Government 2010) also focused on carers' individual rights, introducing the Carers Rights Charter. Carers in Scotland continued to be regarded as contributors to the health and social care system in partnership with paid care staff, and the strategy called for opportunities for training similar to those offered to the paid workforce. It also called for improved provision of information and advice for carers to enable them to carry out their role more successfully. An emphasis was placed on improving coordination between services to facilitate carers' access to support and carers were encouraged to become as representatives on service planning bodies. There was also an emphasis on the promotion of carers' health and wellbeing through increased access to health checks and regular breaks and on training the professional workforce in identifying carers and being 'carer-aware'. A resource for health and social care staff and students, Equal Partners in Care (EPiC), was established to develop knowledge for paid staff about unpaid care with a view to improving relationships between them and foster a sense of partnership (NHS Education for Scotland, 2013). The core principles of EPiC reflected the key aims of the 2010 Strategy: identification of carers; support for them to manage their caring role; enabling them to have a life outside caring; their engagement in planning and shaping services; ensuring freedom from discrimination and disadvantage related to their caring role; and recognising and valuing them as equal partners in care. Because of the UK-wide remit of the DWP, the strategy was limited in its capacity to influence unemployed carers' access to benefits but there was a commitment to improving the take up of benefits and to maximising income through advice agencies as well as to putting pressure on the UK government to increase the level of Carer's Allowance. The Social Care (Self-Directed Support) (Scotland) Act, 2013 was passed, which allowed for self-directed support to take the form of a direct payment, an Individual Service Fund (similar to the Personal Budget in England), traditional service provision or a combination of the three. Local authorities were empowered to offer carers self-directed support. The Act held out the promise of a human rights-based system of social care support and fundamental social work values, although Biziewska and Palattiyil (2022) argued that the necessary resources were not in place to make this a reality.

In Wales, the emphasis on policy implementation was maintained and arguably reached a peak in the 2010 Carers Strategies (Wales) Measure (National Assembly for Wales 2010). The primary focus of this measure was upon bridging the gap between policies and practices in relation to carers. It required the NHS and local authorities in Wales to prepare, publish and implement strategies for carers in partnership with the voluntary sector, private organisations, carers and service users (Welsh Government/ Llywodraeth Cymru 2011). The emphasis was on 'mainstreaming' carers' issues into everyday working practices in health and social care, including the early identification of carers. It provided detailed guidance on what local strategies should cover. For example, information for carers was to be a key element of strategies and the Measure spelled out the range of information that should be included and how it should be communicated. Carers were described as part of the preventive approach to health and social care being developed in Wales through their roles in promoting independence, preventing admission to and delays in discharge from hospital. The measure refers to carers as *providers* of services – indeed, as 'the single largest provider' – and as a 'workforce'. In 2013, the Carers Strategies Measure was revised, and a delivery plan was set up for 2013–2016 but, amid great controversy, the Measure was subsequently repealed with the passage of the Social Services and Wellbeing (Wales) Act in 2014 (National Assembly for Wales 2014).

In Northern Ireland, the *Caring for Carers* Strategy, published in 2006, reiterated the value and importance of unpaid care because of carers' role in reducing pressures on health and social services, to the wider community. Six familiar key themes in the *Caring for Carers* Strategy were: early identification of carers by professionals; information for carers, including information about the health conditions of those who are cared for; training; employment; support services; and specific attention to the needs of young carers and older carers.

Carers and social care reform

At this stage in the development of policies on carers throughout the UK, several recurring themes were evident, although the contexts within which the devolved governments were pursuing these were diverging. In 2014 new legislation in both England and Wales introduced major reforms to social care. In England, the 2014 Care Act repealed almost all previous law related to carers. It introduced a further significant change in the rights of carers to an assessment, which was extended to give carers the right to an assessment of their needs irrespective of whether the care they provided was substantial or regular. A new definition of 'carer' based on that developed by the Carers Trust was widely adopted: 'A carer is anyone who cares, unpaid, for a friend or family member who due to illness, disability, a mental health problem or an addiction cannot cope without their support' (Carers Trust 2022).

This change was in line with the overarching preventive principle of the Care Act, 2014, which was to promote wellbeing. The wellbeing principle was integral to a whole-family approach, which local authorities were urged to support and develop, with evident implications for unpaid carers. The changed position of carers' assessments required a shift in professional practice from the established approach which had privileged the rights of service users over carers and other family members. In addition, local authorities were urged to provide greater clarity about carers' eligibility for support from the local authority as well as information about other sources of support. A further stipulation of the Care Act, 2014 was that assessments of need of people who are supported by an unpaid carer should be 'carer-blind', with the focus on the needs of the individual service user prior to decisions about how those needs should and could be met. At the same time, statutory guidance on assessments also suggested that the support of family and friends should be part of the holistic approach to seeing a person in the context of their social networks. As with the NHS Community Care Act, 1990, the policy lacked the clarity that local authorities sought.

Section 31 of the Care Act 2014 provided and, at the time of writing, still provides for specific services for unpaid carers, which may be as a direct payment. There is an anomaly in the arrangements for direct payments: whereas they are disregarded in calculations of service users' benefits they are not so for carers because the direct payments are defined as earnings. Thus, carers stand to lose their Carer's Allowance or any other means-tested benefit if they are awarded a direct payment (Clements 2016). This rule also applies if a service user employs a relative to provide care, using their direct payment. A further anomaly arising from this rule is that if a service user pays a carer using their direct payment, the carer might be disqualified from an assessment of needs, since assessments are available only to those whose care is not part of a contract of employment. It would be up to the discretion of a local authority to decide what to do in these circumstances. These anomalies are a good indication of muddled thinking in terms of policies on unpaid care and support for carers and demonstrate how decisions that look promising in terms of improving choice and control for one group can have a negative impact on another.

In Wales, the Social Services and Well-being (Wales) Act, 2014 was a major piece of legislation designed to shift the policy focus further, towards a preventive and community-based model, less concerned with specific categories of service users. Controversially, the Act repealed the Carers Strategies Measure, 2010, discussed earlier. The Wales Carers Alliance was strongly opposed to this repeal as it meant the loss of the NHS responsibility to identify carers (Carers Wales 2018). The Social Services and Well-being (Wales) Act was also criticised for having repealed the targeted rights of parents with disabled children to short breaks. In response, the Welsh government made amended the legislation to replicate the parts of the 2010 Measure related to the responsibilities of the Health Boards in Wales. Nevertheless, the dismantling of the 2010 Measure continued to be a source of frustration and disappointment. The Older People's Commissioner for Wales, for example, argued that there would be greater variation in practice with carers because its legal framework was repealed (Older People's Commissioner for Wales 2018). The Social Services and Well-being (Wales) Act changed the legal definition of a carer and as with the 2014 Care Act in England, a carer was defined as a 'person who provides or intends to provide care for an adult or a disabled child' (Section 3(4)). Assessments of need for carers continued to be a separate entitlement and were expected to include questions to ascertain whether a carer was willing and able to provide care and the outcomes they wanted to achieve in everyday life, including whether they wished to take up paid employment or participate in education or training or participate in recreational activities. A national framework for eligibility was set up and a duty placed on local authorities to provide services to meet 'eligible needs'. A Ministerial Advisory Group on Carers was established, and the Welsh Integrated Care Fund was boosted to include additional funds specifically targeted at carers.

Reports from both the Care and Social Services Inspectorate Wales (2017) and Carers Wales (2018) prompted the government in Wales to launch an inquiry into the impact of the Social Services Well-being (Wales) Act, 2014 (National Assembly for Wales 2019). The evidence from these reports suggested that it had not strengthened carers' rights as planned but, on the contrary, had resulted in fewer assessments by local authorities. The first key theme of the report from this inquiry was that although the Act was supportive in its intentions, its implementation had been a disappointment. The finger of blame was pointed at the serious underfunding of the care system but respondents to the inquiry also pointed to the 'dilution' of the Carers Strategies Measure, 2010 which had led the health boards to step back from their responsibilities. They also pointed to the poor level of understanding among front line social workers about carers and about the cultural change envisaged in the Act towards a more strengths-based collaborative mode of practice.

In 2014, the Human Rights Commission of Northern Ireland published a report into the human rights of carers. It identified that there was a lack of awareness of carers' rights, and fears among carers about the future, especially among older carers (NIHRC 2014). They recommended that the Health and Social Care Trusts should be investigated to assess how well they were meeting their duty to inform carers of their rights to an assessment. Betts and Thompson (2016) pointed out that Northern Ireland was lagging behind other areas of the UK in relation to its policies on unpaid carers. For example, while local authorities in England, Wales and Scotland had enforceable duties towards carers, in Northern Ireland Health and Social Care Trusts these were discretionary. The lesson for the rest of the UK, Dayan and Heenan (2019) argued, is that an integrated system does not necessarily produce better results in terms of outcomes in social care or securing new rights for carers. In 2016, the Northern Ireland Legislative Assembly appointed an expert panel to advise on the reform of adult social care services. Their report (Kelly and Kennedy 2017) was hard-hitting, arguing that the Assembly had no option but to introduce radical reform, because the system was in a state of collapse. On carers, the report urged the introduction of similar statutory rights to those in England, so that there would be a binding requirement on the Health and Social Care Trusts to provide support. At the time of writing, there is no legislation but another consultation on social care has been launched.

The Carers (Scotland) Act was passed in 2016 and updated in 2021. It followed a lengthy consultation with carers' groups and was endorsed by the Coalition of Carers in Scotland. It was part of a wider programme of reform, which included the Social Care (Self-directed support) (Scotland) Act, 2013, as well as the integration of health and social care into new authorities. Information and advice became a legal entitlement for carers and were seen as an essential preventive strategy as well as a means of helping carers to negotiate the complexities of the health and social care system. The Act also extended the statutory rights of carers to include those who do not provide care on a 'regular and substantial' basis. As with the Care Act, 2014 in England, this measure was intended to promote preventive interventions and to avoid the pitfalls associated with seeking help only when a crisis has occurred. The term 'assessment' was dropped in favour of the term 'adult carers support plan' as the term assessment was thought to conflict with the idea of partnership in care provision. The change in terminology was intended to encourage carers to discuss their circumstances with a professional and to make it easier for those who were reluctant to do so. Specific adult carers support plans that identified carers' needs and personal outcomes were made a statutory right and the expectation was that these would focus on carers' own perceptions of the outcomes they wished to achieve in life. Importantly, however, to qualify for services, a carer would need to meet the local authority's threshold for support. Otherwise, carers would be given information about resources such as carers' groups.

The Consultation Paper published in 2014 ahead of the Carers Scotland Act, 2016 identified that a lack of clarity existed among both practitioners and carers about the need for a separate carer's assessment. Some carers, such as those caring for a disabled child, it was argued, would prefer a joint assessment of needs and others would benefit from the provision of services for the person they cared for. Although the Scottish government continued to emphasise separate support plans for carers in their own right, they suggested that the support plan could be considered *at the same time* as the community care assessment of the person being cared for. A further duty was that local authorities should consider whether support should be in the form of a break from caring, including whether breaks should be planned on a regular basis. Carers were given no automatic right to a break from caring, but each integrated authority was required to provide a statement on their short break strategy. The Act was followed by the Carers Charter (Scottish Government/Riaghaltas na h-Alba 2018), which reiterated the rights outlined in the 2016 Act and the 2010–2015 Strategy.

Policies on carers' income

An in-depth discussion of policies related to carers' rights in relation to employment and benefits is beyond the scope of this book, but points of particular importance to the overall analysis are discussed here. In 2008, a series of meetings of the Work and Pensions Committee was held to hear evidence related to the government's planned strategy for carers. In her evidence, Imelda Redmond, the Chief Executive of Carers UK, made the pertinent point that while policies on carers had been overwhelmingly the business of the Department of Health, with social services taking on implementation, these affected only a small minority of carers. In contrast, *all* carers were affected by their ability to work or to obtain a decent standard of living through benefits. A large majority of carers, she argued, were of working age but many had to give up work to care and became trapped on a low level of benefits. From these meetings, five outcomes were identified, which informed the subsequent Carers Strategy in England. First, that carers should be respected and valued as care partners by professionals; second, that they should have a life of their own, including in employment; third, that they should not be forced into financial hardship as a consequence of being a carer; fourth, that they should be supported to stay healthy; and fifth, that children and young people should be protected from inappropriate caring. These are largely familiar themes, but the reference to financial hardship is a key issue, largely missing from carers' strategies.

Flexible working

The Employment Rights Act, 1996 and the Employment Act, 2002 first introduced carers' right to ask their employers for flexible working arrangements (Pyper 2018). Flexible working arrangements had been promoted previously in the 1999 Carers Strategy in England as a necessary step in supporting carers and there was a commitment to 'working with employers' to convince them of the business case for retaining employees who had caring responsibilities. The Work and Families Act, 2006 gave all carers of adults (and those who expected to become carers imminently) the right to request flexible working conditions and required employers to consider these requests. This right applied to parents of disabled children and carers of adults who had 26 weeks of continuous service, as long as the person supported was a close relative and lived at the same address. Flexible working conditions could include flexible starting and finishing times, compressed, reduced or annualised working hours, job sharing and working from home. Employees could make only one request per year. Arguably, this was, at best, a partial response to carers' demands for equality of opportunity in employment. A Code of Practice for employers and employees was set up by the Advisory, Conciliation and Arbitration Service (ACAS 2012) and an offshoot of Carers UK – Employers for Carers – was established in 2012 with a view to supporting employers to retain and manage employees with caring responsibilities.

The Coalition government (2010–2016) aimed to extend flexible working to make it normal practice and the Children and Families Act, 2014 extended the right to request flexible working to all employees with 26 weeks of continuous service (Pyper 2018). A report by the Work and Pensions Select Committee in 2018 recommended that the right to request flexible working should apply from day one of employment, rather than requiring employees to wait six months. They also recommended that carers should be allowed five days of paid leave annually when resources allow. This report drew on consultations with carers and referred to carers' fears that prevented them from asking for time off work if, for example, they needed to take their relative to a hospital appointment (House of Commons 2018a). The government put on hold the recommendation on flexible working arrangements and rejected the recommendation on paid leave. In November 2018 an early day motion was introduced to by Sir Ed Davey MP, to amend the Equality Act, 2010 so that carers would have the same rights as disabled people to reasonable adjustments at work. This would have strengthened carers' rights to flexible working arrangements. The motion referred to evidence that 52 per cent of carers are denied requests for flexible working (Hansard 2018). A Private Members' Bill – the Employment (Reasonable Adjustments for Carers) Bill, introduced in 2020, did not progress beyond the first reading. At the time of writing, the intention is to introduce a statutory right to one week's unpaid leave for carers.

Benefits for carers

Until 2016, the DWP set the levels of benefits throughout the UK. Northern Ireland had devolved powers, but reciprocal arrangements ensured parity with the rest of the UK. After the Scotland Act 2016, changes were introduced by the Scottish government as discussed further in this section. In England, Wales and Northern Ireland, the Carer's Allowance, announced in the first Carers Strategy in 1999 and introduced in 2003, has been set at a consistently low level and has been a source of frustration amounting to anger over the years to the present time. In addition, it has been hedged about with limits and qualifications. For example, it applies only to individuals that provide at least 35 hours a week to a person who receives a qualifying disability benefit and to one carer supporting one person. Full-time students have been unable to claim it. In addition, the benefit is withdrawn when earnings from other sources reach a threshold. Carers who receive Carer's Allowance and are employed have been placed in an invidious position, as they stand to lose more than they gain if they receive a pay rise. Carer's Allowance also overlaps with other benefits, which means that claimants lose their allowance when they receive another cash benefit that is higher. This affects carers who qualify for the State Retirement Pension, for example. A British government review in 2010 identified these issues as a problem for carers which had also been raised in the 2008 Carers Strategy. Buckner and Yeandle (2007, 2015) highlighted financial hardship among carers who were on Carer's Allowance and in 2022 Carers UK reported even worse conditions in the context of the cost-of-living crisis for carers on low incomes (Carers UK 2022). As discussed in the previous chapter, evidence of financial disadvantage among unpaid carers has been a consistent feature of research since the 1990s. There is also evidence of confusion regarding the design of the Carer's Allowance and what the payment represents. While some carers perceive it as a form of 'wage' or reward for care work, it was originally designed as a form of maintenance. In their response to the report of the House of Commons Work and Pensions Committee (2018), the government described it as 'a measure of financial support and recognition for people who give up the opportunity of full-time employment in order to provide regular and substantial care for a severely disabled person. It is not intended to replace lost or foregone earnings in their entirety' (House of Commons 2018b). This description reflects a view of caring that might have been expected in the 1990s, with its reference to 'regular and substantial' care, while the low level of benefits also raises questions about what kind of recognition the DWP Committee would consider appropriate for carers and why the benefits system is designed to be so disadvantageous to them.

After 2016, Scotland's approach to financial support for carers diverged from the rest. The Scotland Act 2016 devolved new social security powers, so that the Scottish government has been able to develop its own approach to social security, with the bulk of devolved expenditure relating to disability and carers' benefits (Mackley and McInnes 2020). Universal Credit remains a reserved power with the Westminster government, with some differences in Northern Ireland. Since 2016, the Scottish government introduced a new Carer's Allowance Supplement, which raised the level of carers' benefits to that of the Job Seekers Allowance. A more fundamental change under discussion at the time of writing is to introduce a Scottish Carer's Assistance benefit. Similar qualification rules apply: the carers must be providing 35 hours per week or more to a person who receives a qualifying benefit. However, if a carer is supporting more than one person, they are entitled to an additional sum, currently set at £10 per week. Further changes in preparation are a removal of the barrier to full-time students' access to the Carer's Allowance and the introduction of a Young Carer Grant for those aged 16–18. The Scottish government is therefore making some headway in reforming carers' benefits where it can. Otherwise, the history of policies related to carers' employment and income is striking in terms of the slow pace of change. The low level of the Carer's Allowance is considered by many to be offensive to carers and contributes to a sense of gross injustice that successive policies and strategies have failed to dispel.

Austerity, the COVID-19 pandemic and unpaid care

In 2019, prior to the COVID-19 pandemic, Carers UK sent a briefing to Westminster MPs ahead of an Opposition Day Debate on social care. In this they pointed to the loss of support because of reductions in local social care service provision, which, they argued, had resulted in fewer carers' assessments of need, fewer opportunities for a break from caring, greater use of accident and emergency departments as well as delayed and inappropriate hospital discharges because of a lack of care in the community. The impact of the underfunded social care system on carers was increased isolation and loneliness, a huge strain in juggling work and care, and greater financial hardship, seen especially in those who had been caring for 15 years or more, with higher levels of debt because of having to use their own money to pay for equipment and services for the person they support (Carers UK 2019b). All in all, the picture painted in this Briefing Paper covers similar ground to earlier campaigns by carers, except that the circumstances of carers had worsened considerably because of the impact of austerity policies on services for the individual being cared for.

A Carers Action Plan 2018–2020 in England, *Supporting Carers Today* (DH 2018), continued to draw on the strategy published in 2008 by the Labour government. It contained few new ideas and rehearsed many that are long-standing. At the same time, pressure was building from other quarters about high levels of unmet need in the social care system. The absence of a Carers Strategy by the Westminster government was condemned by Barbara Keeley MP, who pointed to the stresses experienced by carers during the COVID-19 pandemic (Hansard 2021). A White Paper published in 2021, 'People at the heart of care', contained some proposals that were welcomed by carers' organisations (Carers UK 2022a) but there was a strong consensus of opinion that the funds proposed to implement the proposed reforms were far below what was needed (Bottery 2021, LGA 2021).

In 2019, the Scottish government established an inquiry into social care, to which the umbrella body, the National Carer Organisations, responded (NCO 2020). They suggested that for the first time a consensus was emerging across Scotland about the value of social care and the need for change. This, they stated, would require a new social care model, with a sufficient level of resourcing, effective implementation and consistency across the country. They also argued that social care should be envisaged about more than personal care and its role in preventing inequality should be recognised, so that carers could enjoy equality of opportunities and freedom from anxieties about poverty. This document was couched in terms of *rights* to social care, including the right to services to enable them to take up employment and to respite care.

In Wales in 2019, evidence suggested strongly that policies had not achieved the preventive approach envisaged in relation to unpaid care. Llewellyn et al (2022: 94) concluded from the evaluation of the 2014 Social Services and Wellbeing (Wales) Act that there was ample evidence of 'suboptimal' experiences with more negative than positive impacts on wellbeing and a sense among carers that unless they were in crisis, they would not get attention from health or social services. The impact of the COVID-19 pandemic on the implementation of change cannot be ignored but Llewelyn et al suggested that the pandemic also acted as a 'stress test' for the policy and showed in stark relief the importance of social services support for carers. A new strategy for unpaid carers was launched in 2021 (Welsh Government/ Llywodraeth Cymru 2021).

In Northern Ireland the wider political context and lack of stability in government has had a profound impact on health and social care systems, with predictable implications for unpaid care. The 'Transforming Your Care' proposals, 2013, had emphasised the importance of enabling people to receive services at home but in a statement that bore a strong resemblance to comments on the NHS and Community Care Act in 1990, Carers UK Northern Ireland pointed out that while care at home is preferable to care in institutions, without adequate support it will end up being a burden on unpaid carers (Carers Northern Ireland 2013). Their comments were borne out by the 2021 *State of Caring* Report (Carers Northern Ireland 2021), which identified that only 26 per cent of those surveyed had had an assessment in the past 12 months and almost a quarter of them had waited more than six months to get one. In addition, almost a half of carers surveyed said they did not know what services were available.

Unpaid carers are among the groups most affected by the cost-of-living crisis, current at the time of writing. A Carers UK survey (Carers UK 2022b) found that two-thirds of those on Carer's Allowance or on Universal Credit with the Carer Element were unable to meet their monthly expenses. Overwhelmingly, this group of carers expressed anxiety about their finances, a third having fallen into arrears with their energy bills and a quarter having turned to food banks.

Conclusion

This overview of policies and strategies on carers in the UK reflects both continuity and change in policies and in the underpinning principles. When the Carers (Recognition and Services) Act was passed in 1995, the comment was made that its impact would be gradual. More than 25 years later, it is still not clear what the impact has been. Recognition of carers has changed in many respects, especially in terms of carers' involvement in the policy process and service planning. But there is little progress on awareness of carers in other policy areas of direct relevance to them, including other health and social care policies. It is fair to conclude, therefore, that recognition has advanced significantly in some spheres but that it is partial, because it is not yet embedded in other policy areas.

Related to the theme of recognition is emphasis on support for carers 'in their own right' (Lloyd 2000). Over the period under discussion, the trend towards decoupling carers' rights from the rights of the individuals they support has become firmly established and has major implications for practice, as discussed further in Chapter 4. This trend also points to shifts in the balance of responsibility for support between the state and unpaid carers. From the outset, the contribution of unpaid care to the social care system has been understood, but the ways in which it is perceived has shifted as carers have asserted their claims to be perceived as deserving of support in their own right, not merely as an appendage to the individual they support. This has implications for the organisation and funding of services as well as for professional practice. The personalisation agenda, introduced under the Labour government, is a related theme, which has highlighted tensions between the rights of carers and those they support. It also demonstrates how a particular policy agenda can be promoted without due attention to other relevant policies. The low priority given to service users with a carer is a long-standing issue, and inequity in the allocation system for individual budgets demonstrates, as discussed in this chapter, that the capacity of governments to exploit unpaid carers continues unabated, irrespective of carers' improved statutory rights. Information about their rights has featured in all carers' strategies since 1999 as a key factor that enables carers to access support. Yet, many carers remain unaware of their rights and unsure how to access support. Increasingly the focus has been on encouraging health authorities and GPs to take responsibility for giving carers information, on the grounds that they are more likely than social services departments to come into contact with carers during the normal course of their work.

The changing role of unpaid carers in the policy process and service planning is another theme to be explored further. This includes the growth of carers' advisory groups in all governing bodies throughout the UK as well as at local and regional level. The idea that carers are experts by experience is now well established but at the beginning of the period covered in this text it was unheard of. In this sense, the moral case for carers' support is established and widely accepted but the political case for resources to provide practical support is not. Relationships between central, devolved and local levels of government have emerged as another theme. The Carers Strategies Measure in Wales, 2010, was a prime example of centralised controls, with detailed guidance and targets for local authorities to follow. The Scottish government's reforms to financial support for carers demonstrated how differing priorities can be enshrined in policies when powers are devolved from the centre. There are many implications for carers' organisations arising from debates about where decision-making power should lie and what should be the role of carers' groups in decision-making. Carers' organisations have succeeded in gaining access to the policy process in the English and Scottish parliaments, the Welsh Senedd and Northern Irish Legislative Assembly, and have had success in keeping carers' issues on the agendas. Yet, with some exceptions in the devolved governments, there have been few fresh ideas about support for carers in policies and strategies.

These themes will be followed up in subsequent chapters, beginning with a discussion of service development and professional practices in Chapter 4.

4

Policies into practice

Introduction

The focus of this chapter is on the development of services for and professional practice with unpaid carers, primarily in social care. The chapter will continue to explore the themes identified in the previous chapter, by exploring developments in the organisation of services and professional practice at the local level. Key points of discussion involve the tensions and challenges that have arisen in practice since the 1990s, related to professionals' perceptions of carers, the experiences of carers within the social care system as well as their roles in service planning and provision. As discussed, the framework of practice has shifted significantly over the period under discussion. For example, in the early 1990s, professionals and service managers were being urged to take account of unpaid carers' needs when they assessed the needs of service users but since then the focus has moved towards demands to engage directly with carers in their own right. This change in emphasis has generated organisational changes in local authority social services and in their relationships with the voluntary sector, particularly with organisations representing unpaid carers' interests. A focus on the outcomes that carers wished to achieve became a dominant theme in policies and was encouraged as a priority for professional practice with a view to stimulating innovations in support.

Innovative approaches have been a challenge to envisage in practice, however, in the context of resource shortages, and the effects of contradictory policy strands are experienced by practitioners as part of their normal working lives. During the early part of the 21st century the development of specific services for carers was boosted through the allocation of ring-fenced funds to local authorities. When the ring-fence was removed, resources were allocated specifically for work with carers, but the more resources in general were cut, the harder it became to earmark funds in this way. Far from encouraging innovations, therefore, resource shortages have had the effect of reducing the overall level of support significantly. Cuts over the past decade especially have been distributed unequally, leading to additional resource problems for some local authorities, especially those in socioeconomically deprived areas (Yeandle 2016). In addition, the organisational context of provision has been an enduring challenge, as health and social care services have been in a state of almost constant reorganisation, and this has absorbed the time and energy of local authority managers.

Enabling carers to access services has also been an ongoing challenge. In 1999, Banks noted that while carers *in* the system were relatively satisfied with their services, getting access to the system was harder in some local authorities than in others. These inequalities were partially explained by inequalities in carers' socioeconomic background and by the nature of the disability of the person being supported, but variations between services, teams and even individual workers pointed to different attitudes and priorities on the service provider side, which had led to what Banks termed 'the lottery of location' (Banks 1999: 5). Successive governments have attempted to do away with the postcode lottery through central government control, but at the same time they have also pushed for the establishment of local partnerships and corporate bodies whose priorities reflect local interests. The extent of central government control over decisions made at the local level has been an enduring tension in practice. Carers' organisations have been part of this developing picture as service providers and as representatives in local strategic partnerships as well as through their involvement in administering all-party parliamentary groups.

In 1998, the King's Fund, which had conducted a long-term impact study with a view to improving support to carers, published its *Carers Compass* (Banks and Cheeseman 1999; King's Fund 1999), which was intended to be used as a tool in auditing and developing services. The compass was based on eight key outcomes that carers involved in the project had identified as important. These were: full information; recognition (including having their own health taken into account); a life of their own (necessitating quality services for the carer and the person cared for); time off; emotional support; training and support to care; financial security; and a voice in service planning. All the elements of this model have emerged from time to time since 1998 and what carers said was important to them then remains much the same now. In 1999, Banks noted that after 1995 an unnecessarily narrow view developed of what constituted support for carers, which had favoured specialist carer centres, specialist professionals and self-help groups. She argued that existing mainstream services for disabled people, such as home care, should also be regarded as a source of support for carers. In this analysis, Banks hit upon another key tension that has persisted throughout the intervening years, evident in assessments of need, the personalisation agenda and the provision of breaks for carers (respite care), discussed further in this chapter.

Practice Guidance

Practice Guidance is important in shaping service provision, and although it does not carry the force of legal requirement it acts as a standard against which local practice is judged. In 1995 four aims were set out in Practice Guidance to the Carers (Recognition and Services) Act (DH 1996). The first was to move towards greater recognition of carers by 'paying attention to' and 'taking account of' what they say. This can be interpreted as a somewhat meagre interpretation of recognition, as it makes no demands of the practitioner in terms of demonstrating that they have taken account of what a carer says or how they enable carers to articulate their needs and demands. The second aim was for local authorities to make an assessment of the range of care available for service users, but to do so 'without destroying existing informal support networks'. The third aim was to shift practice towards an integrated family approach, which 'does not see either service user or carer in isolation' and the fourth was to improve practice through discouraging bureaucracy and 'providing the opportunity for a private conversation without an elaborate procedure' (DH 1996: 1). This guidance gave ample opportunity for local authority managers as well as front-line practitioners to interpret their responsibilities in different ways and for geographical inequalities to emerge.

According to the Carers National Association report *Still Battling* (Holzhausen and Jackson 1997a), in those local authorities where the 1995 Carers (Recognition and Services) Act was implemented with enthusiasm, there were evident tangible benefits for carers. But the report found that a lack of information was widespread, meaning that carers did not know about their improved rights or about the services that they might have been entitled to. There was therefore an 'urgent need to translate policy at the highest level into practice at the grassroots' (Holzhausen and Jackson 1997a: 44). Robinson and Williams (2002) found that in the case of carers of people with learning disabilities, assessments were still being offered at a time of crisis, rather than as a matter of course, which they argued was against the spirit of the 1995 Act. They also made the point that many people with learning disabilities had never been in the care management system and therefore the essential trigger for an assessment of their carers' needs was absent. Seddon and Robinson (2001) found that knowledge of the legislation was minimal not only among carers but also among care managers. Adequate local strategies were lacking and there were inconsistencies in perceptions of carers' roles as substantial or regular. Some differences in approach emerged between the four countries of the UK. A report on social services departments' experiences of the 1995 Act published jointly by the Carers National Association, the Association of Directors of Social Services and the Association of Directors of Social Work in Scotland suggested that the Act had enhanced carers' access to information, although often at a time of crisis rather than routinely. As was said at the time, assessments of carers' needs at an earlier stage would prevent crises and yield better information about carers' needs (Holzhausen and Jackson 1997b). In Wales, there was a higher likelihood of carers being advised of their new rights under the Act from their GPs and other health professionals. Carers in Wales were also more likely to get respite care (62 per cent against 50 per cent in the UK as a whole). The higher figures in Wales were possibly a result of higher numbers of people in the care system. In contrast, in Northern Ireland, there were fewer carers' assessments, which was explained largely by the fact that there were also fewer assessments of service users' needs.

By 2000, the Practice Guidance to the Carers and Disabled Children Act called for a shift in practice in several respects. Although the legislation still applied only to carers where the service user's needs were assessed, it called for better practice in identifying carers. It also called for improvements in assessment of the impact of the caring role on the carer and support for parents of disabled children was given particular attention in this respect. Other proposals were for innovation in services, a pragmatic and unbureaucratic approach to assessment and a 'holistic and family-based approach' to support, in which carers (and those they cared for) would be seen as *partners* of the practitioners in the caring relationship (DH 2001a). Following the 1999 Strategy for Carers, a multi-agency approach was encouraged, which would involve education, housing and health as well as social services and would mean that assessments could be carried out by staff other than social workers. The idea of partnership with carers and service users reflected a difference in emphasis compared with the 1995 policy, which had been more akin to a traditional service model. This was the case, for example, in relation to direct payments, which were extended to carers, including parent carers and those aged 16–17. Another example was the encouragement to practitioners to adopt a 'positive outcomes focused' approach to the assessment of needs, to assist the carer in finding ways of achieving the outcomes *they* wished to achieve. This is discussed further in this chapter in the section 'Assessments of need and risk'.

In their response to the Guidance on the Act, the Association of Directors of Social Services (ADSS 2001) argued that the Department of Health had seriously underestimated the resource implications of the legislation. In their view, since it had already been difficult for local authorities to reach out to carers, extending services to more carers was unrealistic. They argued that additional services were unaffordable when set against the pressures on budgets. Moreover, they pointed to inequalities in the eligibility criteria that applied to support for carers and those applied to other groups and argued that this generated unfairness in practice between disabled people and carers. In general, while they welcomed the spirit of the Strategy for Carers and accepted the principles underlying the Carers and Disabled Children Act, they argued that without additional resources, the patchy response to the Carers (Recognition and Services) Act, 1995 would be compounded (ADSS 2001). To a large extent, this proved to be the case, as the envisaged whole family approach did not gain ground but care management with individuals continued as the norm in a climate of resource restrictions and an evolving mixed economy of services.

The Social Care Institute for Excellence (SCIE 2007) produced a guide to implementing the 2004 Carers (Equal Opportunities) Act in Social Care. This continued the themes of carer participation in service development; co-ordination and partnerships between the different bodies involved in providing health and social care services; and stronger duties to inform carers about their rights, including the right to an assessment in circumstances where the person they support is not receiving services. Consistent with the contemporary interest in 'evidence based' policies, it included references to research findings on practice with carers and to examples of good practice. Consistent also with the 'network' style of governance espoused by the government, they emphasised the importance of local strategic partnerships of service providers and reinforced the requirement on local authorities to work jointly with health services. In their review of the 2004 Act Seddon et al (2007) commented that limited knowledge on the part of practitioners and a lack of 'ownership' of practice with carers stood in the way of successful interagency and multi-professional practice. They argued that the climate of resource constraints and limited investment in carer services had led to ambivalence among practitioners about carers' assessments and they suggested that specialist staff, or carers' champions, be appointed at the local level to raise awareness and understanding of policies. In addition, they called for greater consistency in establishing carers' eligibility for assessment and for a better understanding among practitioners of the complexity of carers' lives. In Scotland, attention was on assessment of carers and service users in the context of free personal care for older people. Official guidance was that practitioners should take account of the care that a carer is providing, to recognise that care and construct a package of care for the service user as a partner with the local authority. Bowes and Bell (2007) argued, however, that there were differences in the perspectives of service providers on the one hand and service users and carers on the other. Where the former perceived categories of care needs, the latter perceived care needs holistically.

In the sphere of mental health services, the Care Programme Approach also had its critics (Carpenter and Sbarini 1996; Allen 1998; Carpenter et al 2004). Simpson et al (2003), for example, described service users' experiences as consistently disappointing, with carers saying they were ignored by professionals. Haw-Wells (2017) identified a long-standing problem for carers of a lack of information about care plans, which led to a low level of involvement in developing these. The use of jargon by professionals was also discouraging to carers and Haw-Wells argued that a culture shift was required 'so that the carer is recognised as the most important person to the service user from the start of the process' (2017: 56).

By the time of the Care Act, 2014, in England there was a plethora of guidance. This is unsurprising, as this Act replaced the many pieces of legislation on adult social care in force since the 1940s. This policy provided carers with the same level of recognition as those they support, which meant that local authorities should offer a carer an assessment in response to an *appearance of need*, not only when one had been requested. In addition, carers became eligible for an assessment without making a request and irrespective of the amount of time they spent caring. The Act, therefore, marked a major shift in recognition of carers and a further decoupling of their rights from the rights of the individuals they supported. In the case of parent carers of disabled children, the Children and Families Act, 2014 became the legislative framework, a move which was widely welcomed, since it overcame the disadvantage associated with having their needs as carers dealt with separately from their needs as parents. Carers UK welcomed the legislation as it secured the rights and entitlements that had been on their agenda for many years. Drawing on a survey they conducted with local authorities, they argued that the Care Act, 2014 was as a catalyst for change in practice, with better recognition, more prevention and earlier interventions, a refreshed approach to assessment, more meaningful interactions between local authorities and carers, with co-production and partnership working (Carers UK 2015). By 2018, however, their submission to the House of Lords Economic Affairs Committee Inquiry into Social Care Funding emphasised the extreme and unsustainable effects of social care services rationing on carers (Carers UK 2018). Once again, the hopes and expectations of carers were dashed in the context of inadequate resources.

In England, Scotland and Wales carers' involvement in planning services was reinforced in legislation. The Care Act, 2014 in England strengthened carers' rights to participate in developing services, or 'market shaping' as it came to be known. In Scotland, an Implementation Steering Group was set up, with representation from local authorities, health boards, third-sector organisations, carers and others. A Coalition of Carers in Scotland launched leaflets for carers, which explained their rights under the Carers (Scotland) Act, 2016 (Scottish Care Inspectorate 2020). In Wales, the Ministerial Advisory Group on Unpaid Carers and a National Engagement Group had the remit of reviewing the implementation of the Social Services and Well-Being (Wales) Act, 2014. In both Wales and Scotland, co-production networks have been established to promote citizen involvement in service development.

Carers and local service planning

As discussed in Chapter 3, health and social care services have been in a state of constant reorganisation since the 1990s and this unstable context has provoked confusion about areas of responsibility and lines of accountability as well as service users' and carers' eligibility (Jones 2021). In turn, further strategies have aimed at improving co-ordination through partnerships as well as multi-professional and integrated practice. The Social Care Institute for Excellence Guidance on implementing the Carers and Disabled Children Act, 2000, for example, devoted a whole section to cooperation between authorities, arguing that cooperation is essential for the support of carers and that a multi-agency strategy is required, involving health, housing, leisure services and education as well as social services. It was also recommended that training and awareness-raising for staff should be provided across all authorities and that in every local area a senior person should be named as the single point of contact on carers (SCIE 2007). There was a strong case for action on coordination between agencies and professions. The King's Fund Carers Impact study (Banks 1999) had identified how unpaid carers were often the only point of contact between different agencies involved in service provision for the individual they supported. The challenges of partnerships and joint working are many and varied (Cameron and Lart 2003; Cameron et al 2014), which have been evident in the context of support for carers. One such challenge has been confusion in lines of authority and accountability in multi-agency partnerships. If, for example, in the spirit of innovation, a health professional wished to set up a support group for carers, which organisation in the partnership would have responsibility for this and to whom would that professional be accountable when working with carers who were not the patients or clients of their employing authority? The financial and organisational complexity of the mixed economy in social care was not conducive to partnership working.

Olsen et al (1997) made the pertinent point that to be enthusiastic about participation in service planning, carers needed to be sure that their involvement was meaningful. Certainly, the involvement of carers' organisations in local planning networks has become more firmly established, as discussed in Chapter 3. The Princess Royal Trust for Carers, for example, worked with the Association of Directors of Adult Social Services to produce an audit tool designed to help local commissioners to know if their services had produced good outcomes for carers (PRTC and ADASS 2010). In Wales, a Carer Aware project, funded by the Welsh government and run by the Carers Trust Wales and Carers Wales, was established to promote awareness of carers and the involvement of carers in service planning in health and social care systems (Carers Trust Wales 2022).

In addition to developing their partnership role, carers' organisations have also increased their involvement in direct service provision, responding to new opportunities provided by the reorganisations of social care (Yeandle 2016). Alcock (2010) pointed to new opportunities that arose for the voluntary sector in service provision, as a pluralist model of social care was consolidated under Labour governments between 1997 and 2010. Those opportunities have had an impact on the voluntary organisations, however. Means et al (2002) traced the process of formalisation that occurred as a 'contract culture' developed in community care services for older people. This formalisation process involved mergers and rebranding, which enabled carers' organisations to occupy niches in the pluralist system, able to compete with the private sector. For example, the Princess Royal Trust for Carers, established in 1991 to provide carer support services, merged with Crossroads Care in 2012 to become the Carers Trust, which now operates across the UK with multiple functions, including administration of the All Party Parliamentary Group on Young Carers, professional training and consultancy work as well as direct service provision. In Northern Ireland, local groups merged to become Crossroad Care NI. Securing contracts to provide services within corporate partnerships has become an increasingly important income stream for organisations such as the Carers Trust (Carers Trust 2020). Willis et al (2021) identified that more than half of 150 local authorities in England had contracted all their services for carers, including some or all assessments of needs, to third-sector organisations, mostly those working with carers. The involvement of the voluntary sector in service provision has provided local authorities with the means to manage the tension between increasing activity with carers and managing smaller budgets. It also gave local authorities the reassurance that work with carers was being carried out by specialists. This was evident in the Older Carers research project, when one local authority manager, explaining their decision to contract out their work with unpaid carers, said: 'We're not very good at talking to carers or knowing what carers want, and actually our vast majority of our time is on the service user. So, let's give that whole view around carers too, to an organisation that's much more tuned in to carers' (O'Rourke et al 2021, 377).

Certainly, when contracted work is blended with other strands of a voluntary organisation's activities there can be spin-off benefits. For example, in addition to carrying out assessments, carers' organisations offer advice on legal rights and cash benefits; they can inform carers about the support groups they run for health and wellbeing and about how they can get a break from caring. There are also disadvantages to consider, however. Competition for contracts yields negative consequences for those that lose out and often the losers are smaller and less well-resourced than the winners, who have access to professional advice on bidding. This can lead to geographically uneven services, depending on where a successful agency is based. In addition, those that succeed in gaining contracts might find they are obliged to change their preferred way of working to comply with commissioning bodies' demands. For example, Moriarty et al (2015) noted how some local authorities were closing day centres run by voluntary organisations and that when carers' organisations objected to these closures, the local authorities tended to dismiss their views as old-fashioned because they were at odds with their drive towards personalisation. Another example from the Older Carers project was a requirement on a voluntary agency contracted by the local authority to conduct all assessments of need by telephone rather than face-to-face, which the agency would have preferred. Thus, while contracts are a valued source of income, indeed increasingly essential as grants have been cut, voluntary sector organisations might be constrained by commissioning bodies' own priorities. Larger voluntary organisations with multiple functions have been better able to survive the pressures and because they have more strands of work and income, they are better positioned to maintain some control over their activities (Kendall et al 2018).

Perceptions of carers

In Chapter 3 the change in emphasis over three decades towards support for carers in their own right was discussed, with reference to the implications of this change for service provision and professional practice. Twigg and Atkin (1994) commented on the increased visibility of carers in the policy debate during the 1990s but they also pointed to the ambiguities that existed in how carers were perceived in the health and social care systems. These ambiguities, they argued, had led to confusion for agencies in developing practice. Drawing on findings from their empirical research, they developed a four-part model of perceptions of carers, which has been very influential in subsequent research and policy commentary (see, for example, Pickard 2001; Clements et al 2009; Seddon and Robinson 2015; Marczak et al 2021) and is still highly relevant. First, most often, carers are perceived as *background resources*, the 'taken-for-granted social reality against which agencies operate' (Twigg and Atkin 1994: 12). This perception is consistent with a residualist model of welfare, in that seeing carers as background resources leaves the state responsible for stepping in to help only when this form of support becomes unavailable. Twigg and Atkin (1994) argued that perceptions of carers as background resources meant that the state was at best only marginally concerned with carers' welfare and there was no attention given to the potential for conflict of interest between a carer and the person they supported.

The second model is of carers as *co-workers*, where professionals work together with unpaid carers in ways that minimise the boundary between paid and unpaid care. The primary focus of interventions is still the individual supported and the morale of the carer is primarily of instrumental importance. The main concern is with the quality of care. In this model, conflicts of interest are acknowledged but tend to be subsumed under the assumption that carers want to care and should be assisted in doing so. The third model is of carers as *co-clients*. This places carers within the system as individuals who have a need for support in their own right. As such, their eligibility for help becomes a focus of the professional, whose role is to determine whether an individual carer's needs meet the eligibility threshold for support. Conflicts of interest are fully recognised and the problems these pose for the carer become the focus of attention. The fourth model is the *superseded carer*. In this, the aim is to transcend the carer and cared for dyadic relationship via two potential routes. In the first, a disability rights perspective, a disabled person could be free from the need for an unpaid carer by being provided with sufficient services to ensure their independence. Alternatively, from a feminist perspective, an unpaid carer can be relieved of their caring responsibilities by adequate provision of services for the disabled person. Either way, the aim is the cessation – or at least the minimisation – of unpaid care. In this model, the carer and disabled person are perceived as separate individuals, and there is full recognition of the potential for conflict of interest between them. These four models are not fixed entities and individuals in caring relationships might experience more than one at different points in their caring career. The official Guidance on the 1995 Carers (Recognition and Services) Act that practitioners should intervene 'without destroying existing informal support networks' (discussed earlier under 'Practice guidance') reflected the view that informal (or unpaid) care is the norm and that the role of service providers is to keep it going. This approach upheld the background resources model but also contained elements of the co-worker model, in that the Act was intended to give specific attention to carers in an instrumental way.

How carers are perceived by professionals and service providers is key to their claims for recognition. In 1989, Pitkeathley noted that the answer to the question 'what should be done for carers?' is usually along the lines of: 'We should recognise and acknowledge the contribution made by carers. They should be involved in planning services and be treated as full and equal partners, not as mere recipients of services' (Pitkeathley 1989: 125). At that time, in her role as Chief Executive of the Carers National Association, Pitkeathley was an advisor to Sir Roy Griffiths, the architect of the community care reforms. Clearly the aim then was to push for recognition of carers as co-workers – a higher level of recognition than would be the case if they were (mere) co-clients. On the other hand, the view of carers as co-clients persisted. For example, Christine Heron, a commissioning manager and social work teacher, argued that following the 1995 Carers Recognition and Services Act, 'recognition of the role of carers means they are now considered alongside service user groups as a group towards which organisations have a responsibility to provide support' (Heron 1998: 222).

These different perceptions of carers continued to co-exist after Pitkeathley was writing and are sometimes confusing. For example, at the time of the

2014 Care Act in England, Dame Philippa Russell, Chair of the Standing Commission on Carers, wrote:

> At last, carers will be given the same recognition, respect and parity of esteem with those they support. Historically, many carers have felt that their roles and their own well-being have been undervalued and under-supported. Now we have a once in a lifetime opportunity to be truly acknowledged and valued as expert partners in care. (DH 2014)

This lack of clarity about how carers fit in to the system of social care arises partly from the different levels of debate and whether the focus is on individuals or on carers as a whole group but the duality of carers' position as partners (co-workers) and/or co-clients is problematic. How are they to be perceived by others in the care system and what are the implications for the individual being supported by a member of their family who becomes an expert partner with professionals?

Pickard (2001) drew on Twigg and Atkins' model of carers in the care system in her analysis of three policy documents: the National Strategy for Carers (HM Government 1999a), the report of the Royal Commission on Long Term Care (1999) and the Note of Dissent from that report, which arose as a result of differences of view about carer-specific support. While the majority argued that services should be 'carer-blind' – that is, the existence of a carer should not mean services would not be offered – the minority dissenting group argued that more specific help should be given directly to carers. Both groups recommended the provision of respite care (or short-term breaks) but the thinking behind their two approaches differed. The dissenting group emphasised respite care as a carer-focused service, to maintain carers' ability to continue caring and to give the carer 'time for themselves', whereas the majority group's view was that respite care should be understood as a substitute care service for the service user, which also provided relief for the carer, so they would not be overburdened. The Note of Dissent, therefore, chimed with the 1999 Strategy for Carers in its emphasis on supporting carers in their own right, with resources specifically earmarked to this end. While the majority view resembled the 'co-client' model, the minority view resembled a 'co-worker' model. While both approaches were instrumental, in that they were concerned with enabling carers to continue caring, there was greater interest in the welfare of carers per se in the minority, dissenting group, as reflected in the 1999 Strategy. The majority view of the Royal Commission, that services should become increasingly carer-blind, ran counter to this trend as it represented a *substitution* model of services in which carers could potentially be replaced by paid care services. Pickard argued that the main advantage of this approach was that it focused on the needs of both individuals in the caring relationship. The substitution model has obvious cost implications, which in terms of the drive to greater efficiency in resource allocation was – and continues to be – less likely to influence policy makers.

Carers' campaigns for recognition arose from their position as background resources and the language of policies is littered with references to the need for better recognition of their role and contribution. Fears that family ties could be weakened by inappropriate professional intervention have deep roots, as discussed in Chapter 1. The Barclay report on the role of social workers (Barclay 1982) noted that professionals tended to withdraw support from people with unpaid carers either because they *could*, in the knowledge that the person would be cared for anyway, or because they thought the family *should* care, whether they wanted to or not. Arguably, carers are less in the background as resources since their campaigns have raised the level of recognition of their role but as co-clients with service users, they have seen their sources of support shrink during the years of austerity, especially since 2016. The carers as co-workers model approximates to the Scottish government's approach to support for carers, where (as discussed in Chapter 3) support for them was described as 'resources' necessary for them to carry out their function rather than as 'services'. The superseded carer model has been evident throughout policy debates at different points in time, notably in campaigns for direct payments so that disabled people could employ paid personal assistants, on the principle that this would be more empowering than unpaid care.

Identification, identity and recognition

There is an important link between the carer identity and access to services. Up-to-date and accurate knowledge about the local profile of unpaid care is important to local authorities' ability to develop their local strategies and plans for carers and to respond to concerns about unmet needs. Comparison between the numbers of carers counted in the Census and the numbers of carers known to a local authority gives an indication of unmet needs, although this is not entirely straightforward, because not all carers counted by the Census want support from the local authority. In addition, as more activities are contracted to voluntary agencies, local authority data on levels of support becomes less reliable (Fernandez et al 2021). It is estimated that levels of unmet need are high, especially among certain groups, who have become known as the 'hidden carers' (Knowles et al 2016). There are several explanations why some individuals are not identified as carers. Cook (2007: 113) referred to the groups who were missing from the carers' movement, who, arguably, would overlap with those not known to local authority services. These included carers from economically disadvantaged groups, minority Black and ethnic communities, carers with mental health difficulties, older and physically disabled carers, young carers and gay and lesbian carers. Heenan (2000) also identified carers living in rural areas as among those less likely to be known to local authorities and Willis et al (2011) identified the same for LGBTQI carers. Hepworth (2005) and Katbamna et al (2004) pointed to the extreme pressure on carers in South Asian families and the poor understanding of their circumstances by local authorities. Systemic problems can occur in some spheres of practice: carers of people with mental health problems, for example, can miss out on support if they are not the service user's 'nearest relative' (Berzins and Atkinson 2009; Smith 2015; Shaw et al 2018) or if there are concerns about patient confidentiality (Haw-Wells 2017). Older and disabled people have not been recognised by local authorities as carers if they are also service users and some local authorities' records systems are unable to recognise an individual as both a carer and a service user (O'Rourke et al 2021).

Explanations of the 'hidden carer' phenomenon are frequently at the individual level rather than being acknowledged as a systemic problem and underpinned by unwarranted assumptions: 'A significant number of people with caring responsibilities do not readily identify themselves as carers. They understandably see themselves primarily as a parent, spouse, son, daughter, partner, friend or neighbour. The concept of caring is assumed but not recognised in some families in ethnic minority communities' (HM Government 2010: 8). It follows that encouraging carer self-identification has been promoted as the best way to target and support people in caring roles. As Morgan et al (2021) pointed out, without it, carers lose out on financial and practical support but at the same time reluctance to define oneself as a carer can easily translate into being seen as personally responsible for the lack of support. For example, professionals and managers frequently cite the 'problem' of getting older people to identify as carers (Gillies 2000; Lloyd et al 2020). In research with LGBTQI carers (Willis et al 2011) a participant referred to the pathologising potential of language, pointing out that terminology like 'hard to reach' can appear to place the fault on the individual carer rather than the service. General practitioners and other health professionals have been increasingly encouraged to identify hidden carers, because they are more likely than others to encounter carers regularly in the course of their practice with service users (Moriarty et al 2015; Anfilogoff 2018). In addition, employers have been encouraged to identify individual carers in their workforce (Lewis 2016). This drive towards self-identification as a route to obtaining services is open to question, however. It suggests that support for carers is not perceived in terms of what they *do* but on what they *are*, and whether they fit into a bureaucratically and politically defined category of service users. It also removes responsibility from professionals and service providers for noticing carers who might need support. Arksey et al (2003) identified several barriers that had prevented carers from obtaining health care. Professionals were unable to identify carers and were unaware of the impact of caring on health. They had poor understanding of what caring entailed and took little account of carers' ability to attend health appointments or to afford to pay for substitute care. Arksey et al also found that carers' attitudes to their own health and needs caused them to be reluctant to seek help because they had become accustomed to placing the needs of the individual they supported above their own. Arguably these barriers confer responsibilities on service providers and professionals. That health professionals in 2003 had a poor understanding of the impact of caring on health is not easy to explain but that this poor understanding has persisted since 2014 is even more inexplicable, especially given the weight of research evidence and policy activity since then. More importantly, as discussed in Chapter 3, the existing legislation in England, Scotland and Wales places an expectation on professionals to put carers in touch with agencies for an assessment where there is *an appearance of need*. The responsibility has been lifted from carers to ask for an assessment before it is offered and the threshold for a referral is set very low.

As discussed, definitions of a carer have not been consistent in practice. In early policies, when carers were perceived in relation to those they supported, this was not a contentious point. Indeed, the 1999 Strategy (HM Government 1999a) says nothing about the carer identity and in their guide to implementing the 2004 Carers Equal Opportunities Act, the Social Care Institute for Excellence stated that it was '*not sufficient* to rely on carers to identify themselves' (emphasis added). It was recognised that since the term 'carer' might be problematic for some carers, professionals engaged in outreach work should use expressions such as 'Do you look after someone?' rather than 'Are you a carer?' (SCIE 2007: 15). Establishing their distinctiveness as a group has been a long-standing aim of carer-led organisations and, in 2006, a campaign was launched to protect the title of 'carer' exclusively for unpaid carers (Lloyd 2006). This campaign aimed to dispel any misunderstanding that the term applied to *paid* carers and through self-identification it was hoped that carers would avail themselves of the benefits they were entitled to. A campaign to push for wider identification of carers led to another Private Members' Bill, the Carers (Identification and Support) Bill, sponsored by Barbara Keeley MP, in 2007 but this was not enacted before the general election that year (Hansard 2021). In later policy guidance, professionals were encouraged to persuade individual carers to self-identify and to 'come forward' as carers. This was the expectation, for example, in the Implementation Plan for *Caring about Carers* in Wales (National Assembly for Wales 2000) and in the 2010 update to the Carers Strategy in England, 2008 (HM Government 2010).

Willingness to adopt a carer identity is impeded by many reasons as identified in research over years. If individuals do not do so, their chances of being recognised as a carer by professionals are diminished and they run the risk of remaining unsupported. On the other hand, a self-ascribed identity does not necessarily lead to recognition within the health and social care systems or generate benefits or services. In addition, the broader definition of a carer in use since 2014 does not translate into eligibility for publicly funded support. Guidance on the Carers (Scotland) Act 2016, for example, makes clear that while all adult carers are eligible to have a carer support plan, the local authority must provide services only to those who meet a predetermined threshold (Scottish Government/Riaghaltas na h-Alba 2021). The distinction between eligible and non-eligible carers is troublesome because it suggests that the local authority will decide if you are a 'real' carer. This is a prospect that might well act as a deterrent to carers considering whether to ask for an assessment of needs, especially as there is no guarantee of support to follow (O'Rourke et al 2021). The identification of carers has not been a consistent line of policy and it appears that carers are increasingly expected to take responsibility for making known their identity as a prerequisite for attention. The National Institute for Health and Care Excellence Guideline (NICE 2021) emphasised that the 2014 Care Act made it the responsibility of service providers to identify carers, even when carers did not regard themselves as such, although the Guideline also urged practitioners to encourage carers to recognise their caring role and to explain that the benefit of doing so is that their support needs can be addressed.

Assessment of needs and risk

Since 1990, the separation of assessments of needs from the provision of services to meet those needs has been a central plank of care management, as discussed in Chapter 1. When service users' needs were assessed, it was not uncommon in the early years of community care for assessment forms to contain a question related to carers but attention to carers' needs was very limited – hence the finding that they were perceived as 'background resources'. In 2014, after the term 'substantial and regular' was scrapped as a means of establishing eligibility for support, unpaid carers had equal access to an assessment of needs in England and Wales. It had been expected that as a consequence of the Care Act, 2014 there would be a rapid increase in the numbers of referrals for carers' assessments but in 2015 the National Audit Office identified a reduction in carers' assessments and access to services (National Audit Office 2015). In England in 2020 more than half of local authorities had contracted out their assessments to voluntary organisations who also provided services for carers (Willis et al 2021). When assessments identified carers' needs as 'complex', the carers were referred back to the local authorities for further assessment. The definition of 'complex needs' is unclear but it is associated with the interplay of the needs of carers and service users, where meeting a carer's need would require a service for the person they care for or where the health condition of the person being supported demanded more services. In Wales, where most assessments were retained in the local authorities, this organisational complication has not arisen. Here, when assessments are being conducted, a holistic approach is preferred, with the needs of both parties in a care relationship being considered together. If a carer requests it, or if the initial shared assessment indicates a need for it, a separate assessment is provided. In Scotland, the focus has been on the development of Single Shared Assessments, which can be carried out by a local authority or health professional and the carer will be offered Self Directed Support. In Northern Ireland, at the time of writing, carers do not have a right to a separate assessment but are in a similar position to carers in the rest of the UK prior to 2014.

As assessments have always been the gateway to services, it is not surprising that carers' campaigns have focused on assessments for carers in their own right, because this reinforces the perception that carers are no longer an 'appendage' of the service user they support, nor are their needs subjugated to the needs of that individual; indeed, the person they support might not be a service user. The term 'assessment' has been something of a bugbear for practitioners over the years because of its authoritarian overtones and potential to deter carers from requesting help. In the Older Carers project, for example, several assessors preferred to describe an assessment as a 'chat' (O'Rourke et al 2021). It is unfortunate that in the attempt to be less off-putting, practitioners appear to have created confusion, as evidence suggests carers are unsure if they have had an assessment. In Scotland, the off-putting term assessment was dropped in favour of the Adult Carer Support Plan in the hope that this would encourage more carers to identify themselves and to reflect what was regarded as a truer reflection of the aim of the practice. Arguably, this terminology is more forward-looking and potentially a way of linking practical support with unpaid care.

After 20 years of research on unpaid care, Seddon and Robinson (2015) found 'significant and enduring tensions' associated with practice in carers assessments. They identified four main areas of tension: practitioner ambivalence; uncertainty in supporting carers in and beyond their caring role; capturing the dynamics of caregiving and caring relationships; and 'distinguishing between carers' willingness and ability to continue caring' (Seddon and Robinson 2015: 17). In Wales, practitioner ambivalence was related to a lack of clarity about how and why carers should have specific attention within the unified framework of assessment in operation. Practitioners were also keen to avoid any duplication of effort. Seddon and Robinson maintained that practitioner ambivalence had contributed to delays in providing assessments, which meant that they were often conducted at the point of a crisis, as Templeton et al (2021) also identified. Practitioners were also reluctant to pay attention to the complexities of balancing carers' other roles with their caring roles and claimed that the forms used in assessments impeded their ability to capture the carers' narrative accounts of their needs. Attention was concentrated on the tasks of caring, with little interest in the emotional and psychosocial aspects of caring relationships and little attention to the dynamics of the relationship, including planning for the future.

Scourfield (2005) reflected on inadequacies in social workers' practice with carers and argued that a deep-seated problem existed in their relationships, which was largely the result of the idealised views of carers in policies. Moreover, he argued that the perception of carers as 'background resources' was part and parcel of policies, which were bound to create tighter eligibility criteria for services and additional pressures on carers. Social workers were ill equipped to deal with the contradictions and dilemmas that arose in practice, he argued. Certainly, social work with adults (especially older adults) has become more procedural and task-based, on the understanding that it is a low-skilled sphere of practice (Lloyd et al 2014). A further problem identified by Mitchell et al (2014) was that front-line staff sometimes had difficulties envisaging the support they could offer if, for example, a carer's self-defined outcome was to take up education or some other activity beyond the confines of the social care system. The staff were not trained to work within such a holistic view of people's needs. As a result, they argued, staff were reluctant to spend time on carer assessments and avoided the difficulties that these might generate for them. Arguably, the practice in England of contracting carers' assessments to specialist voluntary organisations could address this specific problem, in that carers' organisations are better placed to envisage a wider set of potential outcomes. A disadvantage, not often discussed, is that by doing so the local authorities also remove any incentive to improve their own practice and thus they further entrench its suboptimal standards. The earlier quote from the local authority manager, in which he accepts that 'we are not very good at talking to carers' (O'Rourke et al 2021), conveys the message that that there is no need to *become* good because someone else is doing the talking better. Given the long history of poor and patchy social work practice with carers, it is not surprising that a local authority would take advantage of the opportunity to offer carers a better service, but local authorities have statutory obligations towards carers and, moreover, high standards of practice with service users also demand attention to carers.

Gaining the right to a separate assessment of needs was essential for carers to come out of the background as a resource but research on the impact of the Carers (Recognition and Services) Act, 1995 and the Carers and Disabled Children Act, 2000 showed that carers' entitlement to an assessment was not promoted widely. Many carers remained unaware of it while others did not realise that a social worker had given them an assessment (Carers National Association 1997; King's Fund 1997; SSI 1998; Arksey et al 2000). Reports over the years have been hard-hitting, with references to a shocking lack of attention to carers and poor standards of practice, which have revealed a great deal about the meaning of the term 'background resources'. In their review of care management in Scotland, Stalker and Campbell (2002) found that senior managers identified support for carers as a secondary objective of care management, although most care managers described carers as having an important role to play in the assessment process. Some care managers saw this role as a resource to help the service user but others saw it as entitling them to support in their own right. These findings pointed to carers' random chances of having contact with a professional who was willing to focus on their needs and was clear about how to address these. Seddon et al (2007) identified inconsistencies between and within local authorities in Wales. There was no way of knowing, for example, how many carers had been offered an assessment of needs, because such data as existed related only to assessments that had been carried out. In 2018 the Coalition of Carers in Scotland found only a small minority of carers knew of their rights to an adult carers' support plan and there were inconsistencies between local authorities in their willingness to offer one.

The 'outcomes focus' in practice, referred to in this chapter, became an increasingly important element of assessments, in theory at least. It is somewhat ironic that this was an attempt to draw attention *away* from the initial stage of assessing needs and towards the desired outcomes of a care plan because policies and practices have continued to focus overwhelmingly on assessments at the initial stage. Seddon et al (2007) pointed out that what was meant by a positive outcome was not entirely clear, but a potential one identified was the carer's ability to take up or continue paid employment. Support for carers was increasingly about more than their caring role and designed to enable them to fit their unpaid caring role into their lives. Arksey et al (2007) commented that in 1996 when they embarked on their research programme on 'Outcomes of Social Care', the term 'outcomes' was unfamiliar but over the course of the programme it became a central feature of public sector practice, largely associated with self-directed support and direct payments. Arksey et al (2007) identified four key elements of a framework for practice focused on carers' outcomes: first, quality of life for the care recipient, including their safety, comfort, dignity and independence; second, quality of life for the carer, including health, peace of mind, financial security and opportunities for employment and social activities; third, managing the caring role, including information, practical assistance, emotional support and training; and fourth, service process outcomes, including services that recognise carers' expertise and that are accessible and flexible. A focus on what an individual wishes to achieve in life would take the concept of individualisation a step further from standardised service offers but Seddon and Robinson's 20-year study found that the outcomes focus had not become the normal approach to practice with carers (Seddon and Robinson 2015).

A preference for a non-bureaucratic approach to assessment has been evident in policy debates since the 1990s when it was considered that there was 'no need for an elaborate procedure' (DH 1996:1) but because an assessment can lead to publicly funded services, a degree of formality is unavoidable. In addition, a more formulaic approach has enabled service providers to employ staff with lower levels of qualifications to conduct assessments, because there is less reliance on the exercise of professional judgement. After 2014, with the pressure on to reach out to more carers and to conduct more carers' assessments, a formulaic approach became an affordable option for local authorities. On the plus side, a form-filling exercise can make it clearer to the carer that an assessment has taken place and avoids the situation where carers remain unsure if they have had an assessment, but at the same time, as Seddon and Robinson (2015) identified, a form does not necessarily result in a rounded picture, as there is less opportunity to explore a carer's circumstances, for carers to express these in their own terms and for these to be captured in a more nuanced way.

Assessments of carers' needs have remained instrumental in their focus on the sustainability of the carer role and the level of risk that it might break down if not supported. Yet, despite policies to promote a preventive approach, carers have repeatedly reported that they are at breaking point before they get attention. As resources have become more scarce, voluntary agencies under contract to conduct assessments have become more closely involved in the management of those scarce resources. O'Rourke et al (2021:378) give the example of a voluntary sector chief executive, who commented: '[We] want to have as many carers being triaged as we can [to] identify those more at need, because if we can target people on the cusp of carer collapse, we can help the whole system.' The concentration of attention and resources on carers on the cusp of collapse means that the preventive potential of practice is lost and opportunities for forward planning are reduced to a minimum as attention is focused on present emergencies. In this case, the contracted agency had absorbed the crisis-level management culture of the local authority and focused their attention on keeping the system going.

Conflict in care relationships

One of the areas of focus in the study by Twigg and Atkin (1994) was the potential for a conflict of interest between service user and carer. Scourfield (2005) picked up on this point to argue that because of the idealised portrayal of unpaid care, the complexity of the care relationship is glossed over in policies on carers so that no attention is paid to the potential for abuse or neglect in care relationships. Instead, unpaid care is characterised in policy and practice guidance as wholly benign. Ash (2014) pointed to the dilemmas facing social workers when confronted with suspected abuse in family care of older people, including the fear that alternative care arrangements would be equally bad if not worse. Ash argued that professionals failed to challenge problems in the contexts of practice so that older people were often left in risky situations. Milne (2020) also cited research with older people and their carers that identify physical and psychological abuse as well as neglect. As Milne pointed out, accurate figures are hard to obtain because of the privacy of care in people's own homes, but in a study with family carers by Cooper et al (2008), 11 to 20 per cent reported physically abusing the relative they support and 37 to 55 per cent verbally abusing or neglecting them (Milne 2020: 115–116), and the evidence suggests that as people's health declines they become more vulnerable to abuse, particularly in the context of cognitive decline.

Carers are also vulnerable to abuse. Isham et al (2020) examined female carers' experiences of being abused by the individuals they supported and suggested that there was a need for safe spaces where carers can go to talk about these experiences. Scourfield's critique of the idealised view of unpaid care relationships thus remains highly relevant and points to the need to consider how unpaid care is monitored. Willis et al (2021) found that during the COVID-19 pandemic, only a handful of English local authorities invited carers or service users to get in touch if they felt a need to discuss problems in their care relationship arising from lockdowns, although the increase in levels of domestic violence were openly discussed in the media during this time. The potential for abuse is understood but in the context of unpaid care in people's own homes appears to be difficult for practitioners to address. Instead, abuse has been more often associated with care homes, thus, paradoxically, adding to the pressure on unpaid carers to help their disabled relative stay out of them, or with paid home care staff, which also adds to pressure on relatives. The emphasis on maintaining people in their own homes has been a fundamental principle in policy and practice principle for decades, underpinned by service users' own stated wishes but the evidence on abuse and neglect highlights that leaving carers to cope as background resources is a very risky practice.

Support for carers

In the 1999 Carers Strategy, the concept of support for unpaid carers shifted, so that it was no longer considered *only* in conjunction with services for the service user. At that time, the emphasis was on innovation, and ideas circulated about how local authorities could enable carers to have driving lessons, gym membership or help with housework and gardening. A core aim of the 1999 Strategy was to overcome the problem of individuals in caring relationships becoming 'so inextricably entwined that one individual can have no independence of the other' (HM Government 1999:14). The boost to resources following the 1999 Carers Strategy enabled local authorities to provide more grants for carers' groups, such as self-help, mutual support and social groups. Belonging to a group has evidently helped many carers to feel less isolated and by mixing with others in the same boat, given them access to information and boosted their identity as carers. Groups have enabled carers to give and receive support for little or no charge and are now a core element of carer-specific support.

The distinction between services for disabled and older people on the one hand and support for carers on the other has long been recognised as somewhat artificial, because services for the former will act as a form of support for the latter, as many commentators have observed (Walker 1995; Banks 1999; Parker et al 2010). This distinction has been pursued, however, and has generated tensions concerning the focus of service provision. Seddon et al (2007) noted that in practice there was often a lack of recognition that caring involves two people. This mattered then and still matters because decisions in practice about which one of a caring dyad is receiving services carry over into decisions about who should pay for those services and whether they should be free at the point of delivery or charged for. Manthorpe et al (2019) noted the confusion among policy makers in the House of Commons debating the 2014 Care Bill over whether a service was for a carer or for the individual they support. In the House of Lords, Baroness Pitkeathley called for a clearer distinction between the two, pointing out the possibility of confusion and disputes, and the likelihood that without such a distinction local authorities would act against the aims of the Bill and charge carers for services (Manthorpe et al 2019). Her predictions on the possibility of confusion have proved accurate. The explanatory notes on the 2014 Care Act in England state that support for carers may be met by providing services such as replacement care to the person cared for. In law, however, in all parts of the UK, services provided as 'replacement care' are considered a service to the service user, rather than the carer (Clements 2016a). Because personal care in Scotland is free, there is a difference between Scotland and the rest of the UK, but similar issues arise in terms of the focus of support. For example, free personal care does not cover help with housework for a service user, whereas a carer's individual care plan might result in a service to help with housework that is not charged for because it is a service for a carer. There are rational explanations for this, based on the purpose behind service provision and the rules governing their provision arising from carers' position as partners in providing care, but such decisions appear unfair and run the risk of arousing a sense of injustice.

In their meta-review of interventions to support carers, Parker et al (2010) found little solid evidence that services focused specifically on carers were beneficial, although results related to education, information and training offered the strongest evidence. Thomas et al (2017) conducted a meta-review to update what is known about effective interventions and found mixed results, with no pointers to a standardised benefit to carers arising from specific interventions. Instead, they found, for example, that arts-based therapies and counselling had benefits for carers of people with cancer while carers of people with dementia could benefit from meditation and joining a self-help group. Thomas et al (2017) concluded that contact with other people outside their normal networks was beneficial to carers, irrespective of the kind of activity they were involved in. There was no clear evidence on the benefits of respite care, although the qualitative literature suggests that it is essential to carers feeling that they can carry on. As with Pollock's findings on home care services (Pollock et al 2021), the quality of the provision was a crucially important factor in this study. The conclusions of these two meta-reviews that 'no one size fits all' support the emphasis on individualised approaches to service provision.

Direct payments

In Chapter 3, the discussion of carers' strategies showed the growing interest in personalisation and the extension of carers' right to a direct payment became the primary focus of strategies. As discussed, the personalisation agenda was designed largely with disabled people in mind and commentators have noted how unpaid carers were largely overlooked (Clements et al 2009; Moran et al 2012; Glendinning et al 2015; Larkin and Mitchell 2016). Following the 2000 Carers and Disabled Children Act, carers' eligibility for a direct payment in England and Wales was based on the risk that the relationship might break down if support was not given. The sustainability of the relationship was a key issue. Direct payments for service users, on the other hand, were provided on different eligibility criteria: the individual must be at risk of substantial harm. This gave rise to perceptions of inequities, not unlike those referred to earlier in the context of needs assessment in Scotland. For example, a carer could receive a direct payment to employ a gardener to help sustain the care relationship, but a service user would not, because gardening would not be considered a suitable way of helping those who were perceived to be at risk of substantial harm. Indeed, a request for help with gardening might be interpreted as an indication that a person was *not* at risk of substantial harm. Another difficulty was that local authorities were empowered to charge carers for services, which extended to charges on direct payments. As Leece (2002) argued, when taking account of the value of carers' contributions to the care system, the practice of charging them can be perceived as unethical. Perceptions of carers as either co-workers or co-clients can be seen in tension in this argument. Leece also pointed to the rule that applied at that time forbidding the employment of family members as support workers. The rule was regarded by many as discriminatory towards ethnic minorities, who were more likely to employ family members, and Leece argued that it therefore raised serious ethical questions. Some local authorities made exceptions to this rule on the grounds of equality and human rights.

Breaks for carers

The rhetoric surrounding approaches to respite care has changed since the 1990s, with the term 'regular breaks' or 'replacement care' having been adopted in preference to 'respite', with its connotations of burden and association with temporary entry to a residential care home. Breaks for carers have been a long-standing priority within carers' strategies, as might be expected given the increased attention to carers' rights to a life outside of caring (HM Govt 1999). Arguably, however, breaks for carers still resemble respite. The growth in group activities for carers such as mindful meditation, yoga, pamper days, massage and other similar stress-relieving activities suggest that enabling carers to cope and to carry on is the primary purpose. This is not to suggest that such activities are without merit but to question the central role that these now have in carer support since statutory services have been cut.

Carers' direct payments can be used to employ a 'sitter' to enable them to take a break but there is a difference between replacement care and a sitting service in that the former is a service for the service user and usually subjected to a means test while a sitting service is for a carer and is usually free. Generally, a sitting service is for a short break of an hour or two, whereas replacement care is for longer periods. What the sitter or replacement carer does for the person needing support makes a difference but the many grey areas that have emerged have caused confusion. For example, a sitter might provide an occasional snack for the service user but if they were to provide this on a regular basis it would be classed as replacement care. As resources become tighter, the rules become correspondingly stricter. This quote from a care manager in the Older Carers project highlights the point:

> We used to be told that the sitting service could be a carers' service. It's a sitting service to allow the carer to go and do the shopping or attend appointments or whatever but if [the sitter] needs to provide any element of care whatsoever – which obviously is why there's a sitting service in – then now we're told that it has to go on the cared-for person's support, which means that they will possibly have to pay for it. (Lloyd and Jessiman 2017)

The importance of replacement care was identified by Pickard et al (2018), who also identified a link between access to replacement care and levels of carers' paid employment. Arguably, replacement care is a prerequisite of carers' ability to have a 'life of their own' beyond caring and is entirely consistent with the aims of all the carers' strategies since 2008. Rand and Malley (2014) identified several forms of rationing of replacement care. These included 'deterrence', when carers found the struggle to gain access to services too great; 'denial', when particular groups of carers were told they do not qualify; 'delay', when carers were discouraged by the long waiting times for services; and 'deflection', when carers are referred to other agencies for services. In addition to these forms of rationing, Rand and Malley identified the high charges for replacement care as a major deterrent while service providers were also reducing and withdrawing services, such as day care. As Rand and Malley pointed out, such barriers call into question the value of extending carers' rights. They also support Scourfield's observations about social workers' ambivalence towards support for carers. Marczak et al (2021) also identified examples of replacement services being newly subjected to needs thresholds and financial assessment of the individuals they support. Free support for carers, once universally regarded as a good investment, was at risk of becoming subject to charges. Pollock et al (2021) found that home care services for older people with dementia were increasingly targeted at those in greatest need which meant that many families considered not to be in that category were turning to the private sector instead. The high charges imposed by the private sector agencies meant that those able to employ domiciliary care workers were families with the means to pay. When this worked well, the rewards were significant for both carer and the older person as well as the wider family. As Pollock et al (2021) expressed it: 'home care is about supporting relatives in their caring responsibilities *as well as* providing personal care for persons with dementia' (emphasis added). They argued for a refocusing of services as a collaborative and family-oriented service that acknowledges the triadic nature of care between service users, carers and paid care workers (Pollock et al 2021: 2071).

Seddon and Prendergast (2019) conducted a scoping review on regular short breaks over a 20-year period in Scotland and Wales and concluded it should be a key priority for policy makers as it holds out the possibility of mutually valued outcomes for carer and service user. There were positive impacts on carers' health and mental wellbeing and on the caring relationship, but they also noted that in order for the positive benefits to be fully achieved, the impact of the break on the person being supported also had to be positive. Staff expertise, personalised care and opportunities for medical care were important factors in reassuring carers that the outcomes of a break were good for the person they cared for. A break that does not involve trust in the relationships with the providers of the services used would not benefit a carer. Similar findings arose in research by Cramer and Carlin (2008) in their research on short breaks for disabled children and adults, which was based on a disability rights perspective and strongly focused on the needs of the person receiving care. Research by Greenwood et al (2012) on respite at home for older people with dementia also identified the benefits of the focus on maintaining a sense of normality in their daily routines.

Relationships between formal support and unpaid care

Evidence demonstrates that the lack of services for people who are supported by an unpaid carer lies at the heart of many pressures on caring relationships. Assumptions abound concerning the willingness of older people to continue to care for a spouse, including an assumption that they do not need routine support, despite difficulties arising from continence problems and disturbed sleep. This can be understood as a lack of attention on the part of practitioners but the perception that a service user with a carer is not in 'greatest' need is deeply rooted in policies, which have influenced local service priorities and maintained the professionals' perceptions of carers as background resources.

A particular area of tension between unpaid carers and professionals has been identified in relation to carers' involvement in service users' direct payments. There is considerable evidence to show that professionals assumed carers would manage the personal budget or direct payment of the person they supported. Woollham et al (2018) for example showed that this assumption was common and that in most cases the carers managing the budgets had not received an assessment of their own needs. Turnpenny et al (2021) found parents of adults with learning disabilities had mixed experiences of direct payments or personal budgets, which did not necessarily enhance choice and control. They found that parent carers in their study had to exercise resilience and determination in navigating the care system to obtain what was due to their adult child. Hamilton et al (2017) found that carers of people with mental health problems had to learn to navigate the system and to 'fight' practitioners and agencies to maximise the direct payment. They also noted that parent carers tended to feel excluded and marginalised when care plans were drawn up, while carers who were supporting a partner were more likely to be treated as a unit of co-clients. Coles (2015) similarly identified the conflict and fear that pervaded relationships between the parents of adults with learning disabilities and professionals. In Coles' study, parents appointed as 'suitable people' to manage the direct payments of their sons and daughters felt conflicted by their dual role and unsupported by professionals, some to the point of feeling bullied.

These findings draw attention to hostility in relations between unpaid carers and professionals, which is much harder to explain than professionals' failure to notice carers. Hamilton et al (2017) argued that hostility was borne out of professionals' perception that carers were part of the service users' problems and that a direct payment would help to make the service user independent of the carer. Coles (2015) focused on the power imbalance between professionals and unpaid parent-carers and social workers' exercise of power *over* carers in a hostile manner. The pressure on social workers, whose practice is confined and compromised by the economic needs of their employing organisation, is not conducive to good relationships but is not a satisfactory explanation for such hostility. After all, the professional values of social workers might be expected to generate an interest in the relationships of the service user. Social work values are, however, also rooted in a commitment to individual rights and the promotion of independence. Aiming to support disabled people's rights, some social workers might be committed to a version of the social model of disability that is antithetical to care. Barnes and Mercer (2003: 38) for example, argued that for disabled people '"care" is the opposite of what they want from government policy or service providers, and misrepresents what people need to live independently in the community'. This chimes with the analysis by Hamilton et al (2017) that carers were perceived to be part of the service users' problems.

Explanations of the difficulties professionals have in forming good relationships with carers thus include the organisational, economic and political, as well as the professional and ethical, but evidence over many years suggests strongly that a change in professional practice is needed urgently to counter this problem. Nolan et al (1996) called for practice to be based on a 'carers as experts' model, with an explicit purpose to increase carers' competence. This was a proposed extension of the carer as co-worker model, that involved a multidimensional assessment of needs and a comprehensive range of services and practitioners to assist the carer in developing their skills and knowledge. They suggested a personal, individual approach both to assessment of needs and to reviews of outcomes, rather than standardised measures. In this model the empowerment of carers was the major aim, as it would enable them to see their own needs as legitimate. In addition, Nolan et al (1996) argued, competence in caring would help to overcome the sense of inadequacy and guilt many carers experienced. There are echoes of the 'carers as experts' model in policies that promote training and education for carers and in the practices of voluntary sector organisations that provide such training. As discussed in Chapter 3, the carers strategies in Scotland are inclined towards this approach and resources for carers in Scotland are more generous than in England but the level of resources required to develop practice in the way Nolan et al (1996) envisaged, would be a major barrier to making their vision a reality in the current climate, even in Scotland. Moreover, like the carer as co-worker model it would 'professionalise' unpaid carers with consequences for their relationship with the person they support. A recurring theme in the discussion in this chapter is the absence of attention to care relationships and the dynamic nature of these. For this to become a reality would require even more fundamental changes in practice.

Conclusion

In this wide-ranging discussion of unpaid care and practice in health and social care, the tensions identified are concerning. Yeandle (2016) argued that where the UK used to lead the world in support for carers, it has now fallen behind in many areas. The reflection in this chapter on recurring themes over three decades highlights the ongoing effects of resource constraint as well as of models of care management that value efficiency to the exclusion of other concerns. These effects are evident in services that are inconsistent and practice that is minimalist in terms of its understanding of the complexity of unpaid care relationships. The evidence from research over the decades calls into question the capacity of social services to support carers in developing a life of their own outside of caring, given the lack of an adequate resource base and shortcomings in professional practice. The discussion in this chapter has identified how carers continue to be perceived as background resources but also as co-workers and co-clients. The discussion of practice shows that the aims of policies discussed in Chapter 3 have not been realised in practice and provides empirical evidence of what this means. The next chapter examines the gap between the policy rhetoric and practice in greater detail.

5

Analysis of policies in context

Introduction

The discussion in the previous chapters has pointed to persistent trends in policies on unpaid care over three decades and in practices at the local level. Policies have secured gains for carers but evidently have not delivered what they promised and this chapter examines the gaps between the rhetoric and the reality. Such gaps are frequently characterised as a fault in policy implementation, with explanations focused on the inadequacy of resources or on bureaucratic blockages, which spoil what was originally a 'good' policy on paper. In this discussion, however, implementation is not conceptualised as a separate sphere of activity from policy making. The different perspectives that are brought to bear on how change can and should be brought about to better support unpaid care reflect a complex process of problem identification, negotiation, bargaining and compromise and key aspects of this process are the framing of issues to be included in policies and differences in power between interest groups involved. From this perspective, the inadequacy of resources is a determining factor not only in relation to the implementation of a policy but also in its conceptualisation. A key question raised at the beginning of this book was *why* resources for unpaid care have been so consistently inadequate. A related question raised was why the same demands for better recognition and support have recurred since the 1990s. These questions point to fundamental problems arising from the social and cultural values underpinning policies and the role and purpose of policy making. The distribution of responsibilities between government and individuals when it comes to providing care and support when people need it remains highly contested.

As discussed in Chapter 3, policies on unpaid carers are often ambiguous or opaque, as for example in the definition of a carer in the 1995 Carers (Recognition and Services) Act as one whose role is substantial and regular 'in the everyday sense'. As argued, such ambiguities give rise to diverse practices, 'postcode lotteries' and inequalities between carers which raise questions about the value of policies. There are tensions, also, including a wider, overarching issue discussed by Rummery and Fine (2012), which involves the incompatibility of political aims to meet demands for social justice for unpaid carers on the one hand and ideological commitment to reduce state activities in welfare on the other. In addition, turbulence in the social care system over the decades has given rise to further tensions, as the organisation and management of services shifted towards a corporate model, resulting in changed economic and policy priorities. At the same time, policies to promote individual rights have generated tensions in relationships between rights holders, which continue to be manifest in professional practice. A further twist in this discussion is that since the 1990s research and theorising on policy making and implementation has also changed significantly, reflecting changes in political and economic agendas as well as in the structure and organisation of public services. The reorganisation of public services and the introduction of community care as a mixed economy generated new theoretical explanations and approaches to policy analysis and widened the scope of policy studies. Ayres and Marsh (2014) reflected that over the previous 50 years, changing organisational forms in public services had been a constant theme in policy studies, with differences of view about whether the introduction of markets has diminished the power of the state or simply altered its way of governing.

The imposition of austerity budgets on local authorities and devolved governments highlights the continuing power of the UK government to restrict or undermine the capacity of local authorities and devolved governments to implement their own policy priorities. At the same time, the diversification of organisations at the local level involved in decisions about how care should be provided has demonstrated fundamental changes in ways of governing. As Colebatch et al (2020) pointed out, in the latter part of the 20th century there was a proliferation of 'policy work' occurring in organisations beyond government, including in the commercial and voluntary sectors. An example in the context of unpaid care is the unequal development of policies and procedures within employing organisations on the rights of employees who are unpaid carers. Taken together, these changes pose both opportunities and challenges to carers' organisations, in terms of where they direct their time, resources and energies as campaigners, supporters and service providers.

A historical perspective

A historical perspective highlights the continuities and changes in political programmes over the past three decades and in the cultural values that are expressed through policies. The COVID-19 pandemic revealed, for example, the persistence of ageist and disablist attitudes as well as a continuing lack of awareness of the day-to-day circumstances of unpaid carers. It also raised questions about the purpose and value of policies on discrimination and equality for older and disabled people and shone a spotlight on the organisation of social care services in the UK, revealing more clearly their multiple flaws and weaknesses. The expansion of formal social care services associated with the post-Second World War period had already halted by the beginning of the 1990s (Means et al 2003), but since then, services have been cut to levels unimagined at that time and reorganised in line with the political and economic agendas of neoliberalism. Care has become commodified and monetised, purchased and provided, and the roles and conditions of employment of paid staff have been fundamentally altered accordingly, as have the relationships between paid staff and service users and carers.

A historical perspective also sheds light on the pace of change and the timeframes within which different actors in the policy process operate. Certainly, as already argued, there have been advances for unpaid carers, particularly in *recognition* of their role. Over time, small and incremental changes can add up to a significant difference in the lives of carers and service users. Awareness of carers and of their diversity is greater now than it was prior to the 1995 legislation. Cook (2007: 130) argued that 'in social policy terms [carers] will never be off the agenda'. Yet, Yeandle and Buckner (2007: iv) commented that the recognition and rights gained by carers 'have not yet been strong enough to transform most carers' lives'. The word 'yet' suggests that patience is needed until the transformative impact is realised at a future stage but this observation by Yeandle and Buckner prompts the question to what extent a policy approach that focuses on recognition and rights for carers has the potential to transform their lives. It is important also to clarify the differences between awareness and recognition. Expressions of sympathy for the hardship experienced by carers are two-a-penny but do not amount to recognition that their circumstances represent an injustice. Moreover, perceiving an injustice is not the same as acting to correct an injustice and rights are of little value if a lack of resources or other pressures mean that they are not capable of being exercised. For example, as discussed in Chapter 4, prior to the Care Act, 2014, local authority social workers routinely prioritised service users' assessments of need over carers' because they had a statutory responsibility towards the former. When resources are severely stretched the question that arises is not 'what *should* I do' but 'what *must* I do'? It is not surprising therefore that carers sought parity with service users in rights to assessment but, as Seddon and Robinson (2015) identified, following the Care Act, 2014 that granted these rights, practitioners in England and Wales remained ambivalent towards carers' assessment because they were unable to envisage what support might be available subsequently and were loath to raise false hope among carers.

Not only the pace but also the *timing* of change is elucidated through a historical perspective. Policy makers' interest in carers' demands was stimulated by campaigners' skills in presenting their arguments to fit the wider policy agenda. As Williams (2010) noted, however, carers' claims dovetailed with the shift from institutional to community care at a time when the overriding government concern was to curtail the cost of services. Williams also argued that during the Labour government years between 1997 and 2010, carers succeeded in positioning themselves as 'partners' in the emerging care system and in framing their claims in the language of social inclusion, especially in terms of the barriers they faced in obtaining or maintaining paid employment. As she pointed out, this was consistent with the social investment model of labour market activation, ascendant at the time. Yet, efforts to improve conditions of employment for employed carers has met with only modest success. As Yeandle (2016) pointed out, the UK once led the world in articulating the needs of carers and was the first country to introduce policies to support carers, but that it had lost its leadership position, lagging behind other countries because of the under-resourcing of services and the failure to adopt measures such as statutory paid care leave.

The economic and political contexts

In this section, the policies and practices discussed in the previous two chapters are placed in the context of economic and political developments over the past three decades. An in-depth discussion of the global reach of the neoliberal agenda on social care, although not irrelevant, is beyond the scope of this discussion. The focus is on the context of policy making within the context of the four British governments' approaches to the neoliberal economic agenda and the significance of these to unpaid care. According to Hudson (2021: 11), neoliberalism is 'rooted in the view' that the state is inefficient when compared with the market and that the welfare state had become too large to be manageable. This view underpinned a raft of policies to shift the role of government away from the provision of services to the facilitation of the market. Importantly, the neoliberalist characterisation of the state was that it had become overbearing and paternalistic in its involvement in welfare services, in contrast to the market system, which would uphold individual freedom and choice. At the same time, the neoliberalist emphasis on individual freedom was also expressed in the political agenda to reduce individual dependency on the state and to discourage state intrusion into people's lives. Care given privately in people's own homes with little or no regulation was an ideal means of pursuing this agenda. A further element of the neoliberal agenda, of direct relevance to this discussion, is the way that policy decisions of successive governments have been expressed in terms of a non-negotiable economic reality rather than a political choice. An important observation by Lynch (2021) is that that neoliberalism conflates economic, moral and political understandings, so that economic success and economic probity are framed as virtues. Attempts by the devolved governments to distance themselves from Westminster's enthusiastic embrace of neoliberal agendas over the past decade have been limited in practice by the limits placed on resources.

The market economy in care

The development of markets in social care intensified throughout the UK and became embedded at the local level. At its heart, the political ideology was that the state should be minimally involved in the provision of care and should create the conditions that enable markets to flourish, bringing a spirit of competition, efficiency and innovation into service provision, thus improving its quality. In this context, care provision offered opportunities for enterprising individuals. These changes have had profound consequences for both paid and unpaid care, seen, for example, in the privatisation of the care home market and the insecurities this has introduced for families. For example, the involvement of private equity capital ushered in fundamental changes to residential and home care provision, introducing new forms of risk, such as the unexpected closure of homes when they become unprofitable (Lloyd 2020). Marketisation has been a long-term project, a major aspect of which has been to change local government practices to bring them into line with central government thinking. In 1983, the government set up the Audit Commission to evaluate the economy, efficiency and effectiveness of local authorities in public expenditure (Campbell-Smith 2008). Between 1997 and 2010, the Labour government took this control a stage further with the establishment of the Best Value Inspectorate under the auspices of the Audit Commission. This had a duty to oversee how public authorities were *improving* on the value for money of their services, thus adding inspection to the audit role (Humphrey 2003). Under the umbrella policy of modernisation, the Labour government issued an abundance of guidance, concordats and strategies. The incoming Coalition government introduced their austerity agenda and, ironically, the Audit Commission was itself abolished in 2010, because, according to the Minister for Local Government, it had become a costly creature of the state (Stratton and Pearse 2010). Arguably, since 2010, as a market economy has become further entrenched, the need to audit, inspect and control has reduced because the scope for straying from the central government script has diminished. As a result, the economic agenda pursued by successive central governments has inevitably become deeply entrenched at the local level.

As discussed in Chapter 3, the process of devolution reflected political differences between the constituent countries of the UK, provoking questions about the reach of Labour's modernisation agenda. Williams and Mooney (2008) argued that the governments in Wales and Scotland were not wholly committed to this and that, at least in rhetorical terms, there remained a stronger commitment to welfare based on collectivist principles. On the other hand, as they pointed out, while it is possible to identify differences in particular policies (as discussed in Chapter 3) the overall direction of welfare policies reflected the broader trends evident throughout the UK and at the transnational level. Devolution reduced Westminster's role as the source of policy making and meant that the role of devolved powers was no longer merely the administration of Westminster-based decisions. Newly devolved nations could forge their own social policy path, establishing more distinctive Scottish, Welsh and Northern Ireland measures. In Wales, for example, First Minister, the late Rhodri Morgan, referred to placing 'clear red water' between Westminster and Cardiff (Morgan 2002) and in Northern Ireland, Finance Minister Mark Durkan declared that in relation to policies on partnerships they would not be 'taking a karaoke approach from elsewhere and singing along to it. We intend to develop our own practices and our own approach' (Northern Ireland Assembly 2001). The need to assert a position of difference from England was partly rhetorical but differences of substance also emerged over time, including in social care policies, although these were limited by the low level of resources available. Divergence between the nation governments is easier to perceive in terms of values rather than practices, when the resources required to translate values into practice are lacking.

The significance of this context for unpaid care was apparent in the language of the strategies and in practices within the social care system. From the outset of care in the community, the need for unpaid care has been undeniable and its increasingly central role has been acknowledged in every carers' policy and strategy since. But when examined alongside other, parallel policies, contradictions can be readily identified. For example, Pickard (2010) referred to the contrasting strands in *New Ambition for Old Age*, 2016 and the *Carers Strategy*, 2008. In the former, the emphasis was on choice and autonomy for the individual older person as an active agent while the latter specifically states that the shift to independent living for older people 'will continue to require a greater contribution from carers' (HM Government 2008: 2). This contrast was also evident in the discussion in Chapter 4 on the role of unpaid carers in assisting individuals using direct payments, where the increased independence and autonomy of members of one group were dependent on the assistance of another.

Austerity policies and care

From 2010, sweeping changes were made to welfare spending affecting the whole of the UK, introduced first as part of an emergency budget but in fact designed to reform welfare in much more fundamental ways. These included a cap on the overall amount of cash benefits a household could receive; a limit on child tax credits for families after two children; a freeze on benefits for people not in work and the introduction of Universal Credit to replace existing social security benefits. The cuts were framed as a necessary corrective to the profligacy of the previous Labour government and the promotion of 'responsible politics'. Farnsworth (2021) made the important point that it was not public spending per se that fell during the 2010–2020 decade but spending on targeted areas of welfare. As he also pointed out, austerity *politics* reflected a particular approach to public services, a large element of which, importantly for this discussion, was to promote families as welfare providers in preference to the state. The Coalition government presented this policy as an economic necessity, untainted by ideology, thus reinforcing the inevitability of unpaid care. As Farnsworth (2021) observed, even those who opposed austerity ended up helping to establish it as such. This point was illustrated in Chapter 4, in the reference to a local carers' organisation aiming to target their services at carers 'on the cusp of collapse'. To understand the political point of austerity, he argued, it needs to be seen as a solution not to economic problems but to the welfare state itself. It forced service providers to change the way they provided services if they continued to provide them at all.

Social care services were not a targeted area for austerity, although evidently cuts in the wider context had significant impacts on unpaid care, felt by both carers and those they supported. Brimblecombe et al (2018), for example, pointed to the conflicting aims of encouraging carers to remain in employment while at the same time cutting the very services for disabled people that would enable them to do so. In the run up to the 2010 general election, the Liberal Democrats had pushed for a policy of guaranteed respite care for carers but were unsuccessful. Increased rights for employed carers to request flexible working were matched by a relaxation in the rules for employers, with a greater likelihood that requests would be refused. Many carers were directly affected by the cuts to local authorities' budgets, which led to the closure of services for disabled people (Needham 2012). Similarly, the promotion of preventive approaches in the 2014 Care Act lost ground when the minimum threshold at which service users were considered eligible for services was raised so only when there was 'significant risk' to their wellbeing would they be provided with services. These policy decisions have worked directly against carers' interests and demonstrate how apparent progress in one area of policy can be undone rapidly when the political agenda demands it.

Another major effect of austerity in the UK has been to increase socioeconomic inequalities. According to a report produced by the Equality and Human Rights Commission (Hudson-Sharp et al 2018), the impact of austerity measures was greatest on disabled people, women and children, which has evident implications for carers. Indeed, Carers UK (2014) referred to carers facing a 'perfect storm' of cuts, which came on top of their existing pressures. The cuts to disability benefits and the introduction of Universal Credit had affected the incomes of many carers as did cuts to housing support and Council Tax. After the election of another Conservative government in 2015, the incoming administration doubled down on the fiscal measures of the previous one, with continuing and worsening effects on people in the social care system, including service users, paid staff and unpaid carers, while the cost-of-living crisis current at the time of writing has generated unprecedented hardships.

There has been a profound impact on the employed social care workforce, with lower levels of qualifications and skills required as well as worsening conditions of employment (Glennon et al 2018). Staff reductions and skills shortages have become increasingly common in recent years, while higher-paid skilled jobs at the core of local government functions have been shed to be replaced by low-paid unskilled and insecure jobs. Indeed, Glennon et al (2018) argued that the main challenge for those that remained after staffing levels were slashed after 2010 was to continue to ensure services were delivered at all, despite the pressures of austerity budgets. Corporate management teams with responsibility for service provision were forced to prioritise short-term efficiencies over longer-term planning. Since the early days of the mixed economy in welfare, the complexity of setting clear lines of accountability and fair funding streams in local networks and partnerships has absorbed a great deal of time and energy. Conditions of austerity have exacerbated these problems, placing local authorities in the impossible position of meeting their statutory obligations with grossly inadequate resources. Eckersley and Tobin (2019) argued that austerity policies reduced local authorities' 'policy capacity' – their ability to direct resources and make intelligent, informed choices about strategic alternatives. For example, in the Older Carers project, local authority managers experienced extreme difficulties and uncertainties as they faced a range of local interest groups with competing perspectives and with varying degrees of power and influence over the process (O'Rourke et al 2021). The reduction in spending associated with austerity budgets inevitably had a disastrous effect on discretionary services and adult social care has been a key area of pressure, with local authorities struggling to meet even their statutory obligations.

Governments in Scotland and Wales publicly dissociated themselves from the Westminster approach. MacKinnon (2015), for example, noted a particularly strong emphasis on social justice in both countries. At the same time, as discussed, there were limits to what devolved governments could achieve, given the continued hold of the Westminster government over fiscal policies. Drakeford (2012) argued that for the Coalition government austerity was not a regrettable inevitability but 'enthusiastically embraced as an end in itself', which signalled a striking difference between them and the government of Wales (Drakeford 2012: 457). Certainly, the reductions in spending on adult social care were greater in England than in either Scotland or Wales (Burchardt et al 2016) and Scotland maintained its provision of free social care but as long as social security remained a UK-wide matter, the scope of an independent Welsh or Scottish social care agenda was limited. In their evaluation of the Social Services and Wellbeing (Wales) Act, 2014, Llewellyn et al (2022) referred to the problems of policy implementation where 'historical resourcing and institutional practice issues come face to face with the strains and constraints of the current times' (Llewellyn et al 2022: 57). Those strains included, in Wales, greater demand arising from an older population and higher levels of ill health. In addition, political differences have been muted in practice by the grossly reduced resources allocated from the UK government to devolved powers, leaving them little choice other than to develop social care services as best they could with inadequate levels of funds. Davies and Thompson (2016) described this as 'austerian realism', a term that captures the hegemonic nature of austerity politics. Lowndes and Gardner (2016: 365) argued that austerity politics were a 'neat policy manoeuvre which allows the Conservative government to disavow responsibility for fragmented services it can no longer control, in the context of unpopular and unsustainable budget cuts'. The unpopularity of austerity was recognised and before the COVID-19 pandemic had reached the UK, the Conservative government declared that it had 'turned the page' on austerity. The arrival of the COVID-19 pandemic saw unprecedented levels of public spending, albeit on a temporary basis, including on areas such as unemployment benefits, which previously had been prime targets for cuts but unpaid carers were frequently overlooked and, as previously argued, came under increasing pressure to cope unaided.

The primacy of economic considerations was firmly established in the NHS and Community Care Act, 1990 but shifting public *attitudes* towards markets in care has been a longer term – and arguably incomplete – project. As Pickard (2010) pointed out, old discourses do not disappear but remain as a form of 'sedimentation' underlying new discourses and, as she argued, there is still public support for the collective principles that underpin health and social care policies. The economic and political contexts of policies on unpaid care have been very unpromising and changes in public attitudes towards welfare have also shifted but the values of care, equity and responsibility for others remain and arguably were strengthened during the COVID-19 pandemic.

The policy process

The concept of policy as a process rather than a paper document is now well established in policy studies. The classic but much critiqued model developed by Easton (1965) depicts a staged, linear process through which a problem is recognised as a *social* problem demanding policy attention, a debate occurs over how to solve it, decisions are made about the best solution, policies are finalised and become official, and, finally, are implemented in practice. At first glance, three specific policies to support unpaid carers appear to support this model, in each of which the campaigning and lobbying activities of carers' organisations succeeded in publicising an injustice. Their demands were taken up by MPs, who brought Private Members' Bills before parliament for debate, and thus policies to support unpaid carers were passed into legislation. This process produced the key legislation discussed in Chapter 3: the Carers (Recognition and Services) Act, 1995, introduced by Malcom Wicks MP; the Carers and Disabled Children Act, 2000, introduced by Tom Pendry MP; and the Carers (Equal Opportunities) Act, 2004, introduced by Dr Hywel Francis MP. These three Acts proceeded through a process of implementation with some successes in terms of the outcomes for carers but also with many complaints about the inadequacy of the policies in practice. When examined in historical context, however, it becomes clear that this linear model of a policy process is simplistic. With reference to unpaid care, the next part of this discussion will explore some of the critiques of Easton's classic model.

Debates on implementation

One such critique is presented by Colebatch and Hoppe (2018), who questioned the widely understood perspective on policy as authoritative action – the official version of what governments choose to do or not to do. They also questioned the term 'policy process', in the sense of an ordered unfolding of events from the identification of a social problem to the implementation of the agreed solution. Arguably, such perceptions suggest that policy making is a largely technical, procedural matter and in the case of policy failure generate a search for the point in the process at which mistakes were made. Was there a problem in the initial design of the policy; was the policy too compromised and modified in its formation; were there insurmountable blockages at the local level; was there a failure of leadership; were professionals too intransigent or too poorly trained to bring about change; and – most commonly – was it simply a matter of inadequate resources? Once the concept of a linear process is challenged, however, a different set of questions arises.

An alternative perspective is that the policy process should be understood as a complex web of interests that jostle for attention, who possess more or less power to shape and define the issues under consideration, to influence policy debates and the practices of institutions. Following the groundbreaking work of Pressman and Wildavsky (1984), policy implementation is more often understood not as a final stage in a linear process of policy making but as a determining feature of policy as a whole. The reasons why policies appear to fail are debatable. Indeed, the judgement of whether a policy has succeeded or failed is commonly a matter of dispute: where one interested party sees failure, another sees success. The research by Hervey and Ramsay (2004), referenced in Chapter 4, indicated although the Carers (Recognition and Services) Act, 1995 had limited impact in the short term it generated a shift in perceptions of carers on the part of mental health professionals, so that over time carers became less likely to be overlooked during the process of care planning. Llewellyn et al (2022) argued that the integration of health and social care provision as set out in the Social Services and Wellbeing (Wales) Act, 2014 was difficult to implement because managers in health and social care services needed time to embed the values inherent in the Act and that integration was therefore likely to be a longer-term effort.

As discussed in Chapter 4, joint working arrangements can be experienced as a success by local authority managers if they assist in managerial decision-making, but not by service users if those arrangements do not promote better services. May (2015) argued that it would be a mistake to assume that failure to achieve the aims of policies is a consequence of poor administration or institutional resistance to change. He made the pertinent point that the policy process was complicated by the organisational change associated with the mixed economy of social care provision and shifting spheres of responsibility and accountability, which called into question the utility of diagnosing and correcting blockages in implementation. He argued that such technocratic approaches miss out the *politics* that shape the likelihood of success or failure of policies and that exist from the outset. This observation draws attention to the continuous process of negotiation, bargaining and compromise that make up the policy process and to inequalities in power that exist between the participating groups. The complexity of the social care system, especially when operating within the context of stringent budget cuts, inevitably reduces the capacity of local authorities and their partners and increases the likelihood of counterproductive competition for resources between community groups. A further consideration is that, at times, practice is ahead of policies in introducing innovative approaches to practice. Thus, while a new national policy is working its way through the parliamentary process, groups of practitioners may already be engaged in the process of change it is intended to bring about. For example, in their research on the impact of the 1995 Carers (Recognition and Services) Act, Arksey et al (2000) commented that the local authorities in their study already (to various extents) had local policies in place for carers, and had developed support projects in partnership with local voluntary sector organisations.

Making meaning in policies

A more interpretive approach to policy studies involves asking more of the 'how' questions, including how power is exercised, how the processes of negotiation and compromise work, and how key actors define and respond to an issue. In this approach, policies and practices are conceptualised in essence as an ongoing process of negotiation, rather than a staged process in which practice follows policy making. As already pointed out, the Liberal Democrats compromised on their policy on regular breaks for carers when they became part of the Coalition government in 2010, shelving it for future attention in order to gain a place in government. Multiple perspectives are brought to bear on the process of negotiation and different narratives shape the problem under negotiation. Colebatch et al (2010: 230) refer to the policy process as a process of 'meaning making', drawing attention to the reality that policies do not achieve solutions to problems but settle issues temporarily. This observation highlights the importance to campaigning groups of continuing to keep up the pressure, to ensure issues remain on the political agenda and to influence the way in which their claims are perceived. At the same time, the presence of carers' representatives in policy forums provides a basis for policy makers' claims that their decisions reflect what carers want and need and increases the credibility and acceptability of decisions that are not always to carers' benefit. In the Westminster parliament, debates over carers legislation have generally been very cordial, with a high level of agreement about the value of unpaid care. Indeed, support for carers is widely regarded as a subject above party politics. A typical example can be seen towards the end of the debate on the parliamentary debate on the Carers and Disabled Children Bill, 2000, when Sylvia Heal MP commented: 'We have had good discussions across the parties, which have produced unanimity' (Hansard 2000: c1363). This unanimity settled the issue of carer support temporarily but, as discussed in Chapter 4, was not sustained at the local level, as contradictory pressures became overwhelming.

Implementation is also affected by the interpretation of policy aims. Arksey et al (2000), for example, argued that a lack of clarity in central government aims related to the Carers (Recognition and Services) Act, 1995 led to considerable variations in local implementation, as key actors were able to exercise discretion and interpret the Act in their own ways. This evidence points to Lipsky's concept of the street-level bureaucrat. Lipsky (1980, 2010) argued that front-line workers in public services have discretion over their practice and over the public's experiences of services. However strong the disciplinary procedures over front-line workers and despite restrictions arising from legal and policy frameworks, the capacity for discretion can never be eliminated. Indeed, he argued that inadequate resources and increasing demand for services made it impossible for workers to practice according to expected standards. Hence, the decisions they make and the devices they develop to cope with work pressures effectively *become* the policies that they work to. In the context of resource shortages, local authority social workers are inclined to lower the expectations of service users and to stick to meeting their statutory obligations rather than risk raising expectations that they will be unable to meet (Seddon et al 2007; Ash 2014). Lipsky's insights shed light on the struggles experienced at the local level to establish clear strategies for practice with carers or to generate changes to existing practice.

Differences in levels of power are of crucial importance to the process of making meaning. For example, one of the points of contention already discussed concerns the availability of 'replacement care' services for unpaid carers, which in recent years have become increasingly difficult to obtain. Although carers and service users might complain about the unreliability or poor quality of a service or about the inadequate level of training of paid care staff, provider organisations have an overriding interest in keeping costs down, a viewpoint that coincides with the interests of cash-strapped local authorities. This leaves service users and carers in a weakened position, increasingly grateful for any help they can get whatever the quality, and less likely to complain. Thus, the policies of empowering service users to exercise choice and of enabling carers to take up paid employment are muted by the austerity model that demands low-cost services and is pursued by service providers and planners in line with central government's political priorities. As a result, the market system of social care ends up driving quality down rather than up.

The concept of governance and its critics

The implementation of care in the community in the 1990s, through the promotion of a mixed market, generated significant changes in relationships between different levels of government. This has been described as a shift from vertical to horizontal forms of governance, in which policy implementation is decentralised and placed in the hands of local public, private and voluntary sector agencies, funded by central government and organised semi-autonomously (Rhodes 1997, 2007). The concept of governance draws attention to the weakening of traditional hierarchies of command (Crowley et al 2020). The value of the concept has been questioned because of the many variations in its meaning. Much of the debate centres upon the role of the state and whether there has been a hollowing out of the state's authority and power in favour of the private sector. The governance perspective was embraced by the Labour government as consistent with its radical modernising agenda of local government reform, yet the discussion of the expansion of central government regulation in Labour's modernisation agenda raises questions about the level of autonomy enjoyed by local partnerships and networks. Notwithstanding critiques of the overall coherence of the concept, the governance literature is valuable to this discussion, not least in its perspective on local networks of influence. While all local authorities have suffered severe cutbacks in their general funding and have been forced to withdraw services, they differ in terms of how they have perceived and prioritised unpaid care and carers as well as in terms of how they approached the task of developing support. These variations suggest that local interest groups can exert influence over local service planning and organisation. When an issue is taken up by a voluntary sector organisation or by influential individuals the local impact can be significant, especially in the case of developing partnerships across professional and organisational boundaries. Local groups, such as carers' organisations, typically have a high level of expertise in their specific sphere of practice as well as an ethical commitment to clear goals and ways of working. Their presence in a local network can have a galvanising effect on others and their closer relationship to specific groups of service users gives their practice authenticity.

Service users and carers are, in theory at least, essential to local networks but in practice they might well be overlooked. Barnes (2012) argued that more attention should be paid to the 'rules of the game' operating in local governance systems and to how these should be changed to be genuinely inclusive. This observation draws attention the question of how and under whose auspices local networks form, where and how service users and unpaid carers are involved, who is included or excluded and who has the power to decide? The modernisation agenda of the Labour governments was intended to establish a process of continuous improvement in local governance. After the 2010 general election, the incoming Coalition government continued this agenda with enthusiasm, with a commitment to involve members of the public, including service users and carers, in public services. A new policy initiative, 'Open Policy Making', was developed to this end. What was meant by 'the public' was a moot point. Inequalities in power between participants were evident from the outset of the initiative and there was a strong policy emphasis on promoting the involvement of the private sector as providers, which meant that local networks benefited commercial elites at the expense of less powerful groups. Exley (2021: 463) referred to 'polycentric policy making, diffuse power, new and complex networks ... greater ad hocery and fewer codified rules for participation', which reinforces Barnes' point about the need for attention to the rules of the game (Barnes 2012).

At the same time, although engagement in partnership working is desirable for local voluntary organisations, its effect on them is challenging, particularly if by being more actively engaged in service provision they risk their reputation as campaigners. The participation of carers' organisations in informal local networks has a long history and their expertise is widely recognised but after the implementation of the 2014 Care Act, their position changed significantly, as discussed in Chapter 4. In England, local managers, coping with inadequate budgets were focused on the basic task of getting services to people in greatest need and meeting their statutory obligations, looked to carers' organisations to help in this basic task (Moriarty and Manthorpe 2014; O'Rourke et al 2021). As with voluntary organisations in general, this has meant that carers' organisations have been caught up in the effort to cope with inadequate resources. Ketola and Hughes (2018) examined the shifting roles of voluntary sector organisations in Northern Ireland. When the Labour government was in power in Westminster the voluntary sector had been regarded as essential to peace-building and the development of local governance. In 2010 their involvement became part of the Big Society agenda of the Coalition government. After 2015, however, under conditions of austerity, their role became more closely aligned with the management of scarce resources, which, Ketola and Hughes argued, curtailed their independence and increasingly obliged them to deliver what is demanded of them, in the model of austerian realism described earlier. Many local voluntary organisations have become caught in a bind, facing an existential threat because of the loss of funding but keeping going as service providers under conditions that are far removed from the original principles and values of their organisations.

Framing unpaid care in policies

The following section picks up on the point raised earlier concerning the process of policies as 'making meaning'. The framing of unpaid care is a matter of great importance for policy makers because of the conflicts that arise between different political imperatives. The language used in policies can help policy makers to circumnavigate these conflicts but, as discussed, a lack of clarity in policy documents gives rise to indeterminacy, ambiguity and uncertainty in practice (Smith et al 2019). Unpaid care has been framed in such indeterminate ways in policies, its meaning having shifted between and within policies. The discussion that follows considers three ways in which unpaid care can be framed and considers the implications for policies. Care can be framed as an ideal, as an economic opportunity, and as a social risk.

Unpaid care as an ideal

In Chapter 1 reference was made to the enduring paradigm of the unpaid carer as a hero and to the idealisation of care within families identifiable in policies since the 1990s. The COVID-19 pandemic gave rise to numerous references to carers' unsung heroic status, but this idealised picture masks a more complex reality. Manthorpe et al (2019) tracked parliamentary debates on the Care Bill in 2013 and highlighted how these were conducted without questioning the position of families as providers of care or acknowledging the possibility that carers might wish to reject the caring role. This last point is crucially important. The heroic status of the carers is associated with their assumed willingness to be self-sacrificing. In addition, this framing promotes an ideology that family care is a private activity in which governments should not intervene. A risk attached to this framing is that the competence of the carer is assumed to be adequate. Manthorpe et al (2019) noted a lack of specificity about how carers might be supported or any reference to funding actual services. Worse still, as discussed in Chapter 4, Ash (2014) identified evidence that pointed to the potential for abuse in both directions within a care relationship, particularly where the person cared for had a cognitive impairment. As an activity that is approved of without question in policy debates, unpaid care is rarely considered as potentially damaging to the person cared for. As argued, a heroic status does not invite support, but an additional problem is that it also casts the person who is cared for in a very undesirable light, as passive and burdensome and a drain on the carer. From this perspective, the type of service a carer might want and need is a break from caring and, for this to be a reality, alternative sources of care are required, which meet the needs of the person being cared for. This focus on the needs of both carers and people who are cared for as well as on what supports relationships between them can prevent abuse but necessitates outside intervention in private family life.

Unpaid care as an economic opportunity

Political debate on public expenditure has been infused with concerns about a demographic deficit, arising from perceptions of insufficient numbers of working aged people in the population to support increasing numbers of older people. Debates concerning projected levels of demand for pensions and public services cannot be divorced from policy interest in unpaid care. The Foresight Report on the 'Future of an ageing population', for example, signalled support for families and unpaid carers as a priority for policy action. Actions recommended included helping unpaid carers to balance care activities with other competing responsibilities, particularly work, to meet the increasing demand from the population of people aged 65 and over (Government Office for Science 2016). From this perspective, as discussed in Chapter 3, unpaid care is framed as an economic necessity. A twist on this perspective is to reframe support for unpaid care as an economic opportunity.

The framing of unpaid care as an economic opportunity was evident in policies during the Labour government years between 1997 and 2010 and carers' campaigns at the time featured the business case for support (Williams 2010). In their report on *Sandwich Caring*, Carers UK (2012a) called for the stimulation of care and support services as part of a national economic growth strategy and for improvements in practice among employers through raised awareness of the business benefits of family-friendly workplaces. In this report, the marketised system of care was presented as an opportunity, instead of a confusing obstacle, and care services were described as enabling carers' participation in employment, rather than as supportive to service users. Similarly, in their 2012 report *Growing the Care Market*, Carers UK commented: 'The demographic tsunami facing our society raises the spectre of an unmeetable demand for care requiring a bottomless pit of investment in public services. However, if we turn this around and look at addressing supply it enables us instead to identify the benefits of investment in the care business' (Carers UK 2012b: 8). Indeed, they argued that with increasing demand for care and without a similar increase in supply in formal care, it followed that unpaid care 'surely is *the* inevitable growth sector – a good news story for struggling economies' (Carers UK 2012b: 9, original emphasis). The view that unpaid care can be framed as an economic opportunity gained ground and there was increasing attention to its financial value (Buckner and Yeandle 2015). The perception of care work – both paid and unpaid – as low status belies its value to society but also misses the point that investment in services could benefit the economy by freeing up unpaid carers who wish to participate in paid employment. When it comes to identifying the funds needed to sustain unpaid care, however, a different set of priorities prevail, which relegate care to the status of a cost rather than an opportunity.

Unpaid care as a social risk

The concept of social risk underpins much of the system of welfare established after the Second World War, the introduction of 'national insurance' against the loss of earnings associated with retirement, sickness and unemployment being a clear example. Disability or job loss, for example, carry the potential for poverty and environmental exclusion and these contingencies were understood to be shared by the population as a whole (Means and Smith 1998). New social risks have been associated with emergent employment practices, the insecurities and low wages associated with the gig economy being key examples, and have tended to be seen in relation to specific groups. With a particular focus on unpaid care for older people, Fiona Morgan has presented a lucid argument for unpaid care to be defined as a social risk, that is, as a contingency that is potentially damaging to the wellbeing of individuals affected and which place the risk-bearers at further risk, such as poor health, poverty and diminished career opportunities (Morgan 2018). Unpaid care differs from other social risks in that there are two inter-related risk-bearers: the carer and the person who needs care. Moreover, as she pointed out, each of the two risk bearers has the potential to exacerbate the risk faced by the other. Morgan questioned whether the Care Act, 2014 in England, which granted unpaid carers the right to an assessment on the same terms as those of service users, had indeed recognised unpaid care as a social risk, but she concluded that the Act perpetuated inconsistencies in access and entitlements to services. She predicted correctly, however, that the impact of austerity measures would overshadow any shift of perspective in the legislation and that it would make little concrete difference to carers in practice. In their analysis of the impact of the Care Act 2014, O'Rourke et al (2021) picked up on this discussion to support Morgan's argument and to point out that in practice, the emphasis was on supporting resilience and self-help among carers as well as on avoiding any additional costs to local authorities associated with services for carers. The discussion of unpaid care as a social risk is followed up in Chapter 6, when some of the wider implications of Morgan's analysis are considered further.

These three ways of framing unpaid care indicate the opportunities and pitfalls of campaigns on behalf of carers. The dead hand of austerity is highlighted in all three, associated with increased pressures on, but decreased support for, unpaid carers.

Unpaid carers' rights in policies

Calls for recognition have been a feature of carers' campaigns from the outset, including recognition of their knowledge and expertise by professionals, recognition that solidifies their identity within the health and social care systems, and recognition of their role and what it entails in public life. Campaigns for carers' rights *as carers* have been central to ensuring policies acknowledge these. Given the tendency for their interests to be overlooked and for them to be taken for granted as 'background resources' in practice, this is unsurprising but, as discussed in Chapter 4, a focus on the rights of one half of a caring relationship has not apparently produced a satisfactory outcome.

According to Parker and Clarke:

> [I]n the desire to support informal carers, policy makers have gone down a road that, no matter how long it is travelled down, will never take policy to a position where disabled people and their families and friends can make real choices about how and by whom support is provided in the community. (Parer and Clarke 2002: 348)

Parker and Clarke (2002) argued that despite the success of the carers' movement in becoming centrally involved in the policy process, government support for carers remained problematic. They questioned whether with all the attention that carers had gained, there had been any improvements in core services, such as personal care or domestic help, which, they claimed, were evidently the best form of support for carers. From this perspective, then, the rights agenda for carers had been a mistake because it did not deliver the practical support they needed. The point raised by Parker and Clarke (2002) two decades ago encapsulated the tension that exists to the present day about where the focus of attention should lie in policies. An additional consideration is that when unpaid carers are made the focus of attention in specific policies there is a risk that they will be overlooked in other relevant policies. The absence of references to unpaid carers in policies other than those specifically designed with them in mind is a common phenomenon, even when the policy under discussion is directly relevant to carers. For example, a report for the Social Care Institute for Excellence on social care past, present and future (Wistow 2005) barely mentioned unpaid care. The 'principles of social care reform' set out in this report refer fleetingly to carers only as an adjunct to service users. Perhaps most surprising of all is that this report was written in 2004, the same year as the Carers (Equal Opportunities) Act was passed, when it might have been expected that carers' rights would be at the forefront of thinking. Unpaid carers are now more likely to be considered in the wider policy agenda than in 2004, but their needs and rights are still not evidently in the mainstream of policy debates on social care. At the time of writing, such attention as there is on social care is on its cost and how it is paid for.

Changes in the language of the carers strategies discussed in Chapters 3 and 4 highlight the development of the emphasis on specific rights. While early strategies emphasised supporting carers to enable them to continue their caring role, later ones focused on carers' right to a life outside of caring and consolidated the carer identity, not only in the context of providing care but also in employment and in local community life. Clements (2016a: 5), for example, argued that the Care Act in England, 2014 represented evidence of a 'major cultural shift taking place in the way carers are viewed'. The Carers (Equal Opportunities) Act, 2004 and the Work and Families Act, 2006 were also key to this cultural shift, as discussed in Chapter 3, and over the subsequent ten-year period, Clements argued, carers came to be seen as having a right to an 'ordinary life'. Campaigns for carers' rights and the high priority given to the recognition of carers in policies in countries such as the UK contrasted with the policy emphasis on relieving 'caregiver burden' in North America (Rummery and Fine 2012). At the same time, evidence suggests that the rights agenda has not brought about the desired cultural shift. Azong and Wilińska (2017), for example, examined the framing of unpaid care in the Equality Budgets in Scotland between 2009 and 2014. The Equality Budgets were part of the Scottish government's mainstreaming strategy on gender, which followed the United Nation's Beijing Declaration from the Fourth World Conference on Women (UN 1995). The equality agenda in Scotland and elsewhere was heavily focused on labour market participation and Azong and Wilińska (2017) argued that this focus had negative consequences for unpaid carers, because being outside the labour market, they were perceived as a problem to be managed rather than as productive citizens. They also identified that there were *no* references to unpaid care in the Equality Budgets between the years 2013 and 2015. In their view this was because there was insufficient attention to structures and relationships of power so that other interests eclipsed those of unpaid carers. Thus, the Carers Rights Charter of 2010 did not have the impact envisaged because of competing priorities and perspectives.

Carers have expressed their claims in terms of fairness and justice and in policy debates there is no hint of disagreement with their claim to be recognised within the health and care systems. As discussed, parliamentary debates in all parts of the UK are peppered with references to the hardships endured by carers and to their case for support on the grounds of fairness and justice. At the same time, as Clements (2016b) pointed out in his discussion of the Care Act in England, 2014, no legal rights granted to carers could materialise unless they were adequately resourced. The achievement of new rights in the Care Act 2014 thus held out the promise of fundamental change in the way that carers were viewed but parity of esteem with service users has proved to be of dubious value in the context of austerity. The political priority given to controls over social care expenditure reinforces Parker and Clarke's point about the fundamentally problematic nature of support for carers. Attempts to reconcile the conflicting pressures between reductions in public expenditure and the promotion of support for unpaid carers end up with unpaid carers being characterised as both a cost and a benefit, with the cost perspective becoming dominant as austerity reduces the capacity of local authorities to manage their statutory obligations. A further point to consider is that campaigns for recognition are often about securing the statutory *right* to recognition, in large part to overcome professionals' tendency to take them for granted. As discussed in Chapter 4, several reasons can be given for this tendency, including the pressure that professionals are under and the long-standing practice of one-to-one professional relationships with service users in health and social care services. The demand for separate rights and equality of treatment is understandable in the context of carers' experiences of unfairness but the right to recognition has not been enforced.

Campaigns for improved rights for carers in the context of paid employment are also problematic. If carers succeed in their campaign for caring to be made the tenth protected characteristic under equality legislation, employed carers will have the right to demand reasonable adjustments to their working conditions. This would be an advance over their current right to request flexible working conditions. However, as James (2016: 479) argued, employment policies are often framed by a focus on the economic and business case and improved working conditions are 'often shelved or diluted' when perceived as a burden on business. The impact of such weakness in employment rights is not felt equally between carers. Carers of working age who spend more hours on unpaid work and fewer hours in employment are more likely to be in poverty and those in the lowest paid jobs are less likely to be granted flexible working conditions. And if caring is made the tenth protected characteristic, what would this mean for caring relationships? Concerning the rights of unpaid carers, Clough (2014: 133) argued that there is a fundamental problem with a one-dimensional approach to rights, which is not capable of appreciating or resolving 'the complex interplay of interests inherent in the caring relationship'. Moreover, as Clough pointed out, the law has failed to uphold carers' rights to exercise choice over whether they wish to take on responsibilities for care – a fundamentally important right. It follows that they are also unable to set boundaries over the time they spend in care activities or the tasks they are willing to take on. As research has demonstrated, carers often find themselves becoming carers with little or no discussion about their choice (Arksey and Glendinning 2007; Rand et al 2019) and, as Manthorpe et al (2019) identified, this was not an issue for debate in the run up to the 2014 Care Act, as discussed in this chapter.

Conclusion

In this chapter, the discussion of policies on unpaid care has considered the economic and political contexts that have determined the direction of policies on unpaid care over the past three decades and underpinned their core values, which have been inextricably linked with a neoliberal economic agenda. The turbulence experienced within social care organisations over the same period can be understood by reference to this same context, raising questions over the value of policies on care when these are constantly undermined by the lack of resources. The discussion has focused on the gap between the rhetoric and reality of policies and examined this through the lens of the policy process, in which the meaning of policies is understood as subject to different, often contradictory, perspectives. The concept of governance, with its explanation of policy networks, provides a lens through which to understand the roles of carers' organisations at the local level. The risks to these organisations of becoming incorporated into dominant political and economic agendas has also been identified. The discussion also focused on the framing of unpaid care in the policy process and how different frames reflect inequalities between the groups involved. Unpaid care is consistently framed as an unqualified good in policies but this idealised view belies the potential for conflict between individuals in caring relationships and enables policy makers to avoid questions concerning the need for resources to provide practical help and support. Unpaid care as an economic opportunity has also been part of the policy agenda, particularly during the Labour government years, but this perspective has been eclipsed by the more enduring characterisation of care as an economic cost, especially during the past decade of austerity. The framing of unpaid care as a social risk has potential as a basis for reframing unpaid care with its attention to its widespread nature and the logic of pooled responsibility for its funding. The rights agenda pursued by carers' representatives within the policy process as the way to obtain recognition has had partial and limited success but continues to be a core aim of carers' campaigning. A discussion of this dimension of the policy process is continued in Chapter 6.

This analysis of policies has identified issues that concern the relationship between the state and the individual. That unpaid care can be seen to have served a political and economic project to minimise the activities of the state as welfare provider and to reduce expenditure on social care is undeniable. In addition, the cost of this service to the individuals involved has become increasingly untenable as the crisis in social care is experienced by individuals and families. But this does not tell the whole story, because while support for unpaid carers and services for service users have been cut, individuals and families have continued to care for their older and disabled members and organisations of carers have continued to provide support. The next chapter explores the ethical and political dimensions of care and their relevance to policies on unpaid care.

6

The political and ethical dimensions of care

Introduction

The discussions in the previous chapters have identified shortcomings in policies and practices on unpaid care, not only in the gap between policy rhetoric and practice realities but also in the framing of unpaid care and its place within the wider political context of a marketised system of care. In this chapter, the discussion returns to the point raised in Chapter 1, when Andrew Dilnot said on the BBC's *World at One* programme that it required 'courage and strength of will' to develop policy on social care because it is a subject that politicians would prefer to avoid. Politicians have made enormous assumptions about the willingness of family members to take on caring roles and have also idealised care in the family as a warm and superior option in comparison to formal care services. Policy debates have shown widespread acceptance of the *moral* case for support for unpaid carers and legislation has raised hopes of a cultural change on the horizon which will include justice and rights for carers. Yet, when it comes to developing practical support, unpaid care appears to be persistently stuck as a low priority for state support. As discussed in Chapter 5, the political and economic contexts over the past decade have been unsupportive to the point of destruction to social care in general and to unpaid care specifically. Campaigns of and for unpaid carers have produced copious amounts of evidence and have argued their case at the heart of policy making in all governments in the UK, gaining all-party support. Yet, despite successive policies and strategies to support carers and despite the efforts of campaigners over decades, pressure on unpaid care has increased rather than decreased and while the COVID-19 pandemic brought the gross shortcomings of the social care system to the attention of the public, there has been no apparent change in the direction of policy since. Indeed, in England reforms to social care look set to be resourced inadequately on precisely the same economic grounds as previously, with the added bitter irony that the pandemic is given as a major reason why resources cannot be found. The persistent lack of resources raises questions about the purpose of policies and meaning of rights when these rights amount to such limited practical benefit. Why is it that unpaid care is thought to be capable of infinite expansion, becoming increasingly complex and demanding, but with decreasing levels of support? Arguments that resources are insufficient to provide for care and support reveal not a *failure* of policy but, as argued in Chapter 5, *de facto* the policies on care. The widely held perception that better social care services are 'unaffordable' is deeply embedded, creating the conditions in which those who need care can be characterised as a burden on the economy and those who provide care can be characterised as heroic, especially if they are unpaid.

Policies thus reveal how human vulnerability and the need for support and care are understood and demonstrate the power of a political agenda to shape public perceptions of care. A key question to be addressed, therefore, is why so little consideration is given to the quality of life of people in need of support and care. The distinction between the carer and the individual they support is frequently blurred – indeed, that is part of the heterogeneous nature of unpaid care – and a further question arises about the value of policies that focus on one half of a caring dyad. A major focus of the discussion in this chapter is on the relational character of unpaid care. The discussion will provide a critical view on the ways in which policies have played a part in shaping ideas about care and will present alternative conceptualisations of care and the implications of these for policy decisions on unpaid care specifically.

Unpaid care: a widespread activity or a distinctive category?

In previous chapters, two important perceptions of unpaid care were identified. On the one hand, unpaid care in the UK is characterised as widespread and diverse and on the other hand as distinctive in nature and applying to a specific group. Both perceptions have been evident throughout the period under discussion in the policies discussed but there is an evident tension between them. The discussion in Chapter 2 on the history of research on care pointed to the expansion of knowledge about the extent of unpaid care as well as the diversity of unpaid carers and caring circumstances. That unpaid care is a widespread activity is underlined by calculations about the likelihood of any individual becoming a carer during their lifetime (George 2001; Zhang et al 2019). As Zhang et al (2019) identified, the likelihood of becoming a carer is unequally distributed between population groups based on geography, gender, age and other factors, but their key point was that most people in the UK will be unpaid carers at some unpredictable point in their lives. Indeed, the title of George's publication – *It Could Be You* – was a reminder of the unpredictability of finding oneself in a caring relationship. It was a call to sit up and take notice and not make assumptions that unpaid caring was someone else's business. Moreover, policies and strategies on unpaid care have frequently been introduced with a reminder about how caring affects all of us. Of course, the carer population is not stable; people become carers and their caring roles come to an end. This 'turnover' is also a reminder that a lot of care involves helping people at the end of their lives (Lloyd 2004). In contrast, when unpaid carers first began to be involved as a pressure group in policy-making forums, the emphasis was on their shared identity and their distinctiveness, especially from paid carers and service users. This was necessary for their consolidation as a campaigning group, with their aim set on coming out of the background. As Bytheway and Johnson (1998: 247) expressed it, during the 1990s 'the archetypical question was no longer "who *provides* care?" but "who *are* the carers?"' (original emphasis). Their campaign for recognition was and is still a claim for social justice borne out of their exploitation and marginalisation but the emphasis on their distinctive identity – essential to their claims for recognition – is hard to reconcile with the alternative emphasis on the widespread and diverse nature of care and the likelihood of any one of us becoming a carer during our lifetime.

As discussed in Chapter 4, the imperative to define unpaid carers as a distinctive group also underpins their eligibility for support and services and establishing a distinctive and recognisable identity is therefore a bureaucratic requirement as well as a campaigning imperative. This process of firming up the identity of a carer has led to inconsistencies and contradictions in policies. For example, at the turn of the century, strategies for carers were regarded as being the business of *all* government departments on the basis that carers' identity was more than that associated with their caring activities and that they should be supported in their life *beyond* caring. Yet, notwithstanding recent increased activity within health services, support for carers has been overwhelmingly the business of social services departments, which reach a minority of them. This contradiction also created problems for professionals whose role is to assess carers' needs and develop care plans with open-ended possibilities for what carers wish to achieve in life, while practising within departments under pressure over resources. At the same time, in these processes of clarifying the identity and entitlements of carers, no voice was given to the person *receiving* care. In this way, the carer became socially constructed as an overburdened individual who needed respite from their abnormal circumstances and the conditions were set for the reaction from disability rights activists discussed in Chapter 2.

The ethics of care school of thought conceptualised care not merely as a widespread activity but as a fundamental element of human life. This perspective focuses attention on the social and cultural frameworks of policies and on the values that underpin political decisions. Particularly pertinent for this discussion is the tension that arises between rights and justice on the one hand and care and relationality on the other. The observation by Herring (2014), discussed in Chapter 2, that it is only by understanding human dependency and vulnerability that we can truly appreciate the importance of human rights, is a key point. Evidently, human rights are not a guarantee of protection from oppression and discrimination, although they set a standard against which actions and experiences can be evaluated, as Milne (2020) argued. A major weakness is the lack of attention to the rights of both carer and cared for and the potential for conflicts between them. Milne (2020) also argued that in the context of dementia, the human rights agenda with its individualistic approach contradicts the *relationality* of people's lives. Drawing on Tronto (1993), she argued that the human rights agenda continues to be overshadowed by the wider political agenda of resources. As an example, she cites the 2017 report of the UN Convention on the Rights of Persons with Disabilities, which described the UK's policies for disabled people as a 'human catastrophe' (UN 2017, cited in Milne 2020: 126). Evidently, human rights are not immutable, especially in the face of political and economic agendas that characterise care as an unaffordable cost. The emphasis by Milne (2020) on the relationality of people's lives is crucially important because it points to the contentious relationship between the agendas of justice and care. Thus, declarations of human rights are valuable for articulating public standards and principles, but the policy infrastructure needs to engage with abuses of power, evident in breaches of disabled people's human rights, including in care settings and in their own homes. Human rights exist within political contexts, which determine how those rights are exercised, breached and defended.

Tronto (1993) argued that the perceived boundary between justice and care was based on a false conceptualisation of care as *particular and drawn out of compassion* in contrast to justice, which is *universal and drawn out of rationality*. In her view, 'a theory of care is incomplete unless it is embedded in a theory of justice as well' (Tronto 1993: 166–167). This observation by Tronto can be linked to the point made by Herring (2014) concerning dependency and human rights. From their different perspectives, both Herring and Tronto conceptualise theories of justice and care as interlinked. Kittay's views on the distinction between power and domination are highly pertinent here also (Kittay 2011). As discussed in Chapter 2, in her view, inequality in power is inherent in care relationships where one person is dependent on another, but this inequality is compatible with both justice and care. Indeed, it is the inequality in power between carer and cared for that necessitates an ethic of care to prevent domination and the abuse of power.

As discussed in Chapters 2 and 4, the occurrence of abuse within unpaid care relationships sometimes evokes a weak and ineffective response from professional social workers, and a reluctance to intervene in private care arrangements. This can be understood as an individual failure to recognise an older or disabled person and to uphold their human rights, but Ash (2014) also pointed to the organisational, policy, cultural and moral contexts of practice, which can enable or even encourage professionals to ignore, or fail to see, abuse. Taking account of the perspective of the care recipient, therefore, provides a fuller understanding of relationships of care and the conditions of caring as the contexts within which rights have meaning in practice.

What are the implications of these conceptualisations of justice and care for carers' campaigns for recognition and rights? The policies examined in previous chapters have, as argued, focused heavily on the recognition of carers and have (in theory at least) gradually expanded their rights and improved recognition. A key point concerns the policy focus on carers without reference to the people they care for. In a similar vein to Milne (2020), Barnes (2006: 150) argued that '[b]inary distinctions between rights and care and those which separate care providers from care-recipients do not reflect the fluid identities and experiences of those involved in caring relationships'. Such binary distinctions can be damaging to relationships. Beckett (2007), for example, pointed to the potential for care to be both liberating and disempowering to a disabled person. Drawing on personal experience, she focused on how marital relationships are perceived if one partner is disabled. There is an assumption of inequality within the relationship, with each partner seen separately as a giver and a receiver of care and the two-way flow of care and support that occurs in a relationship is therefore disregarded. Superficially, this perspective appears to be at odds with that of Kittay discussed earlier. While Barnes (2006) and Beckett (2007) perceived interdependencies and fluidity in the giving and receiving of care, Kittay perceived a need to face the realities of dependency. As she explained, her daughter's disabilities have caused her to be 'fully dependent' with little likelihood that her dependence will change much. This, she argued, means that 'it is only with care, and care of the highest quality, that she can be included, loved, and allowed to live a joyful and dignified life' (Kittay 2011: 52). She also emphasised that it is not that her daughter does not reciprocate at all but that the reciprocation is in 'a different coin', in the joy and love that she gives. Moreover, she argues that understanding dependency as an aspect of human life is essential to overcoming fear and loathing of disability. Kittay's perspective therefore is not at odds with Beckett's. Moreover, it has implications for recognition not only of carers but also of disabled people.

Given contemporary dominant social and cultural values in the UK, changing attitudes towards dependency and the need for care is a tall order. The promotion of independence is arguably *the* core value of social care policies, although what this means to the range of actors within the policy process is a moot point. Some service users seek independence through purchasing formal services to avoid becoming a burden on their families. Independence was a strong value in the development of direct payments, perceived in terms of control over support services, which were separated conceptually from relationships of care. Others seek independence through reliance on the family to avoid being a burden on the state. The care of family members can be experienced as a bulwark against the risks involved in being cared for by 'strangers', especially when this involves personal or bodily care. The link between increasing proportions of older people in the population and changing dependency ratios has contributed to wholly negative perceptions of dependency. The association of old age with dependency and burdensomeness is deeply entrenched in dominant political and economic models, to the detriment of older people for whom any acknowledgement of a need for support and care can lead to a sense of being a burden. Unpaid care within families can help to sustain the illusion of independence but being considered – or considering oneself – as independent, when actually dependent on a family member for support and care is paradoxical and can be interpreted as a facet of the invisibility and exploitation of family carers. Dependency is therefore experienced in very different and complex ways, but policies play a major part in framing care and creating the conditions that underpin reluctance to ask for help (Lloyd et al 2014).

Those conditions include the introduction of a market system in social care, which increasingly is understood as a source of additional risk for those who use it and those who work within it. This can be understood by reference to the concept of precarity (Butler 2004), which has been a recent development in gerontology and is of direct relevance to the discussion in this chapter (Grenier et al 2017, 2020; Fine 2020). In a similar vein to that of the feminist ethicists, vulnerability is characterised as inherent within human life, and commonly intensified in later life, but the concept of precarity emphasises how vulnerability is compounded by the marginalisation and devaluation that arises from conditions in which people age, including in the system of social care. Later life, especially when the capacity for self-care is diminishing, brings a heightened sense of precariousness which can be alleviated or exacerbated by social and economic conditions in which people age. As Grenier et al (2020) observe, the concept of precarity is typically associated with earlier stages of the life course, particularly in relation to insecure and low-status employment (Standing 2011). But earlier life experiences also shape and define the conditions in which one ages so that the inequalities and insecurities of earlier life are carried on into later life. Indeed, as Arber and Ginn pointed out in 1992, those on lower earnings are likely to face a heightened risk of illness and disability *and* the inability to alleviate the effects of these because of their lack of material, financial and cultural resources. In a marketised system of social care, these risks are arguably greater because the loss of collectively organised services favours those who are socioeconomically advantaged, leaving those without resources even more reliant on families to support them. As Grenier et al (2020: 1) observed, 'responsibility is now placed on individuals and/or their families to secure support for many of the vulnerabilities associated with old age'. Unpaid carers are thus inevitably caught up in this situation of precarity through their own life course because their caring roles place them at a disadvantage in the labour market and because they rely on services in the social care system to enable them to set limits on their own caring responsibilities, and to 'have a life of their own'. The circumstances of many unpaid carers fit the description of insecurity, poverty and low social status that is also applied to paid care workers, who epitomise the 'precariat' described by Standing (Armstrong and Armstrong 2020). These developments in gerontology amplify Kittay's conceptualisation of 'nested dependencies' (discussed in Chapter 2) and clarify the link between socioeconomic conditions and the experience of dependency. This link is not only about the lack of support in the social care system but also about the way in which the provision of support can *increase* the precariousness of dependency.

The importance of placing socioeconomic conditions at the heart of policy analysis is underlined by Fraser (2009), who argued that both recognition *and* redistribution are crucially important principles for campaigns, which should focus on the structural dynamics of power. In Fraser's view, a politics of recognition is essential to overturn the impact of disrespect and marginalisation experienced by groups on the grounds of their identities. The invisibility experienced by unpaid carers is a result not only of the private 'behind-closed-doors' nature of their role and relationships, but also because professionals evidently do not perceive a relationship of care and carers are thus unrecognised and relegated to their 'background resources' position. It is unsurprising that unpaid carers feel aggrieved over being unseen and undervalued in this way. A stronger resource base is an essential prerequisite to recognition. Indeed, without additional resources, recognition would simply result in carers becoming *foreground* resources, in which their contribution is well understood and appreciated but not supported in practical ways.

A further question to consider is the extent to which recognition is important to different carers. In Chapter 5, the discussion focused on attempts by local authorities to persuade reluctant carers to come forward and identify themselves as carers to obtain access to services. The apparent resistance or indifference to the carer identity considered in that discussion would suggest that recognition is not a top priority for some carers. In addition, it is not altogether clear how the term recognition applies. Are carers demanding to be recognised as a distinctive group, recognised for what they do, recognised as partners with professionals, or a combination of any or all of these? The following extract from an interview with an assessor in the Older Carers research project illustrates the point: '[Older carers] may need things like someone to do the shopping ... strip the beds, help with cleaning. And we can't put that in place. It's frustrating. You would have to fight tooth and nail to get money for that' (Jessiman and Lloyd 2018).

This example raises an important question about whether the primary concern, as perceived by the assessor, is for older carers to be recognised as carers per se, or for older couples whose health problems have compromised their ability to carry out practical tasks to have assistance to enable them to remain together at home. Would the provision of services reduce or remove the sense of indignation expressed by carers and soften their demand for recognition? A focus on such examples highlights the importance of resource distribution as well as recognition. Sayer argues that 'expressions of equality of recognition which are not backed up by equality of treatment and distribution of resources and opportunities are likely to appear hypocritical' (Sayer 2011: 211). Policies that emphasise recognition for carers can end up with fine words about carers' heroism but in the absence of practical support definitely appear hypocritical. In Sayer's view, recognition should be about recognising someone's moral worth as a person, rather than in terms of their identity (Sayer 2005). This is an important point to bear in mind when the diversity of caring circumstances is considered. Sayer also pointed out that the provision of resources is a mark of recognition of an individual's moral worth: the two are inextricably linked. Identity politics can end up with groups competing for a larger share of the purse without questioning the political decisions that imposed limits on the amount available in the purse to be distributed.

The routinisation of care services

In this section, the focus shifts to the political agenda and its capacity for undermining care and shaping perceptions of need and dependency. Waerness (2001) referred to the shortcomings of neoliberal policies for their narrow, economistic focus, which have aggravated rather than solved problems for those who need care as well as for care workers. She pointed to the language of welfare reform, its economic, technical and legal nature, which, she argued, was far removed from the actual world of care. This point echoes the arguments of Twigg (2000) discussed in Chapter 5 concerning the way that the 'bodywork' of care was sidelined in policies that focused upon managerialist and professional concerns. In fact, bodily needs are referred to in policies where the monetary value of personal care is under consideration, such as the Scottish government's policy on free personal care discussed in Chapter 3 where personal care is expressed in terms of itemised bodily requirements (Bowes and Bell 2007). These itemised requirements are used in assessments to determine service users' eligibility for free personal care, which are a bureaucratic necessity for policy makers intent on prioritising efficiency. They also facilitate the marketing of care as a commodity, often with standardised time slots allowed for different items (Seddon and Robinson 2015). What these lists miss out, of course, is any account of *how* an individual is assisted with hygiene, eating, walking or medication. Although services are generally monitored for quality standards and customer satisfaction, a fundamental aspect of care is missing, which pertains to the relationship between the individuals involved. Knowing an individual well enough to be familiar with their preferences, likes and dislikes is part of this relationship. An example can be seen in this account from a research interview in the Older Carers research project, where a care manager is talking about a cognitively impaired man who has his lunch served by one of a team of home care workers when his wife, who is also his carer, is having a break.

> The home care staff don't know him. So, when they ask him if he wants lunch and he says 'no', they just leave it at that and don't give him anything to eat. But I know if you say to him; 'I'm going to make myself a sandwich. Do want to join me?' he will. And he enjoys it. (Lloyd et al 2020)

The relational dimensions of care differentiate it from mechanically delivered services. Lanoix (2013) refers to 'thickly embodied' care, which is responsive to the person being cared for as opposed to 'thinly embodied' care, which is pre-programmed. The provision of publicly funded care has become increasingly pre-programmed and at the same time categorised as unskilled, which affects not only the incomes and working lives of paid carers but also the experiences of those using care services, who become objectified when their needs are met in this 'thinly embodied' way. There is also an effect on unpaid carers, when the services that enable them to take a break are delivered in this way. The carer in the previous example would have returned home from her break to a hungry husband and had to make up for the deficiencies of the service. Arguably, the higher the priority given to efficiency in public services, the greater will be the pressure on unpaid carers to make up the deficit, thus calling into question the value of services provided to enable a carer to take a break. Moreover, when care is reduced to a commodity in service provision, it is easy to contrast it unfavourably with the idealised version of care in the family presented in policies. In turn, as discussed in Chapter 4, families are placed under more pressure to find ways of keeping their relatives out of the care system, in a kind of contemporary version of the Victorian principle of less eligibility. In reality, without adequate support, far from being an ideal, unsupported care relationships are more likely to be a source of pressure, frustration and conflict and the perception of carers as 'background resources' has allowed such pressures to be ignored. Moreover, as Twigg and Atkin (1994) observed, when carers became 'engulfed' in their role, they would be more likely to defend the privacy of their relationships, thus reducing the likelihood that they would ask for help.

This takes us back to the discussion of the relationship between socioeconomic inequalities in the conditions of unpaid care (Arber and Ginn 1992). Moreover, because of the savage reductions in public service provision in the intervening years, the scenario that Arber and Ginn developed 30 years ago is even more pertinent today. Lynch (2021) identified the ways in which the care deficit under neoliberalism is unequally experienced, including socioeconomic and class inequalities in access to services and the gendered and racialised characteristics of care services. An additional point is that the location of support for carers within social services departments adds to the association between support for unpaid carers and social need. The framing of unpaid care in policies has reinforced a perception that it is class–neutral, but evidence demonstrates the opposite. The stigma associated with social services has been identified as one reason why unpaid carers were reluctant to come forward for help (see Chapter 5), although an increased role for the NHS and GPs in identifying unpaid carers could go some way towards addressing this problem. Whether support follows identification depends on the level of resources available in health services and the level of priority given to unpaid care.

The care deficit

The concept of the care deficit discussed by Lynch (2021) underlines Fraser's (2009) argument about redistribution as a crucial element in campaigns for justice in unpaid care. The care deficit can be understood as a description of the gap between rising demand for care and falling supply of publicly funded care but also as a critique of the impact of neoliberal economic agendas on family relationships. Despite the strength of the moral case for support for carers' recognition, the case for resources to support carers has never gained purchase and in the contemporary political and economic context is unlikely to. Tronto (1993) argued that the moral agenda of rights and the political agenda of resources should be understood not as separate but as deeply entwined. Indeed, she argued that the division between the moral and political agendas meant that 'the concerns of the relatively powerless are omitted from the central concerns of society' (Tronto 1993: 20). The ageing of the baby boomer generation was in plain sight when political decisions were made to shift what was at the time health care, free at the point of delivery, into means-tested, marketised social care services, and to expand the role of unpaid care. Political interest in unpaid care and its importance as a means of managing the increasing demands of an ageing population has been quite openly expressed, as discussed in previous chapters. An important observation by Michael Sandel is that markets do not only allocate goods but also 'express and promote certain attitudes towards the goods being exchanged' (Sandel 2012: 9). Cuts to publicly funded welfare and the introduction of a market culture in care have not only reduced the quality of life of those who relied on services but have also shifted public expectations and attitudes about the state's responsibility towards people who need care, with the result that individuals and families have increasingly taken on unpaid care out of necessity rather than choice.

Hochschild (2003: 214) identified different conceptualisations of care that have circulated in debates about the care deficit and how it could be addressed. The first is the 'traditional model', in which the unpaid carer provides nurturing, warm and loving care. Calls by politicians to adopt an 'Asian' approach to care for older relatives have strong overtones of this understanding of care (see Butler 2013; Asthana 2017). Hochschild (2003) argued that this conceptualisation, in which 'caring about' is intrinsic to 'caring for', has become increasingly difficult to sustain. She observed that changed working conditions and increasing rates of divorce have led to higher rates of female participation in employment outside of the home, which have made it increasingly impossible for women to be carers and homemakers in the traditional sense. The second conceptualisation, the 'postmodern model', takes women's participation in employment as capable of being reconciled with unpaid care responsibilities. In this conceptualisation, the mother who 'does it all' became a standard to be emulated. Again, employment conditions work against this model because, for most men and women, there is little or no flexibility that would make employment more conducive to family life. In the UK, as discussed in Chapter 3, although a growing number of employers sign up to carer-friendly practices, the voluntary approach to support has produced unsatisfactory outcomes and carers are still campaigning for paid care leave. Solutions may be sought in technology, with telecare facilitating what Hochschild (2003: 220) calls postmodern stoicism, in which the care deficit is defined as a psychological issue, requiring individuals to manage their needs to fit minimalist norms of care. The third conceptualisation is the 'cold modern' model, which relies on institutions to substitute for family life and address the care deficit in a managerialist way, with a view of care that is rational, practical and efficient, accepting the realities of modern life. This model has been associated with, for example, Soviet regimes but can also be linked to the commodification of care and task-based contractual relationships. There are similarities between Hochschild's cold modern approach and Lanoix's (2013) 'thinly embodied' version of care described earlier.

The fourth model, 'the warm modern', is a mixture of the cold modern in that some degree of formal care is expected but is blended with the warmth assumed to come from family care. In this model, the care deficit is addressed through changes in the structure of work that allow for both men and women to participate in care at home with flexible time schedules at work. In this model, a higher value would be placed on care. How the balance of formal and informal care should be determined is a moot point, but Hochschild (2003) argues for strong co-ordination *between* interest groups, including paid and unpaid carers, to achieve better recognition and an upgrading of their social status. She also argues that the impact of this on the person being cared for would be relief from the sense of being a burden. Hochschild's (2003) model, although drawn from experiences of work and family life in the US, has resonance with the depiction of care within the British context, also. For example, political interest in telecare as a means of managing older people's care needs, helping them to remain in their own homes for as long as possible, resembles Hochschild's (2003) 'postmodern stoicism'. It is regarded as a potential solution to the stress placed on employees with caring responsibilities, enabling them to be 'caring from work' with minimum disruption to their employers' schedules. Telecare is also held up as a solution to carers who live at a distance from their ageing parents. A criticism of her line of thinking, however, is her minimalist attention to those on the receiving end of care. Her depiction of the warm modern approach touches upon an important issue – the potential relationship between paid and unpaid care – but it is open to question because within it the social status of disabled and older people is perceived as reliant on a 'trickle-down' effect from the improved position of paid and unpaid care workers.

With a focus on old age, Kröger (2022) drew on theories of the care deficit, including Hochschild's, to develop his concept of care poverty, which he defined as 'the deprivation of adequate coverage of care needs resulting from an interplay of individual and social factors' (Kröger 2022: 28). In Kröger's view, neoliberalism inevitably ends up with care poverty. Lynch (2021) similarly pointed to neoliberalism and the 'anti-care culture', in which social relations based on risk and reward calculations encourage competition in relation to material wealth, social status and moral worth. She argued that rising levels of socioeconomic insecurity feed suspicion and resentment between people and undermine the trust that is essential for social solidarity and care for vulnerable others. Thus, Lynch (2021) argued, although care is essential to capitalism – indeed it could not survive without it – capitalism devalues care by placing it in a dichotomous position with highly valued economic production. As she expresses it, the exploitative capacity of *homo economicus* contradicts the logic of *homo curans*.

Implications for care policies

The next part of this chapter will focus on the implications of the foregoing discussion for care policies and systems. As discussed, from Tronto's perspective on human dependency and need for care to Butler's (2013) conceptualisation of the precarious life, a powerful case has been developed for the interdependency of human beings. The centrality of caring to all lives is a reminder that care provision is a matter for everyone, not only for those who are categorised by a public system of social care as carers or dependants. From this perspective, care is no longer a private matter confined to the home but a public concern and a subject for political debate and policy action. Key to the debate and action are ease of access to support as well as equity and justice within the system of support.

Katz (2020) considered the idea of the precarious life in relation to critical intersections in the human life course. Unpaid care can be understood within this frame; the 'sandwich generation' of middle-aged women, the 'young carer', the 'young adult carer' or the 'older carer', each group being freighted with cultural meaning and each facing heightened precarity in their own way. As Katz (2020) pointed out, precarious conditions have also given rise to the idea of resilience; the capacity of individuals to bounce back at times of adversity (Donoghue and Edmiston 2020). Rather than bouncing back, the idea of resilience in care services has come to resemble Hochschild's concept of postmodern stoicism, discussed earlier, in which politically and economically induced precarity is characterised as a *psychological* issue, with the expectation that individuals will reshape their needs to fit minimalist norms of care (Hochschild 2003). This quote from an interview with a commissioning manager in the Older Carers research project illustrates the point neatly:

> For me the huge priority is making carers more – I mean, they're phenomenally resilient. They're probably the most resilient group of people that we have in the city, but actually we need them to be more resilient or to recognise things to do, coping mechanisms, earlier, to look at maybe wider family support etc. (O'Rourke et al 2021)

In this vague and somewhat desperate way, the manager is looking to carers to find 'things to do' to enable them to absorb yet more responsibility for the care of people who are about to lose their services. It is notable that this interview took place before the COVID-19 pandemic, at which point expectations of resilience in unpaid care reached even higher levels. As Katz (2020) noted, rather than a solution to the precarious nature of life, resilience becomes part of the problem because it psychologises and depoliticises vulnerability. We might also consider the pressure on carers to identify themselves as carers in this light also, because it entails a requirement on them as individuals to see and define themselves differently, to take responsibility for their own ability to cope with a caring role through support that might be theirs if they do so.

A focus on the conditions of precarity associated with contemporary market capitalism runs the risk of conjuring up an earlier golden age and it is important to re-emphasise that the purpose here is not to romanticise the post-war welfare system but to point to losses associated with its dismantling, as discussed earlier in relation to the care deficit. When human life is understood as inherently precarious, the potential advantages of pooling risks become clearer. In their analysis of individual, or personal, budgets in England and Australia, Needham and Dickinson (2018) argued that the Australian National Disability Insurance Scheme (NDIS), which was based on a system of pooled risk and social insurance, had key advantages over the British system of individual budgets, which had emphasised the purchasing power and choice of a minority of disabled people. These advantages included the peace of mind that comes from risk pooling, its equity and inclusivity and its disassociation from welfarist approaches to support for disabled people. The principles of the NDIS were seriously undermined by political decisions to reduce its coverage and tighten eligibility criteria, but the Labor government elected in 2022 plans to reset it (D'Rosario and Lloyd-Cape 2021; Dickinson and Kavanagh 2022). The NDIS was introduced by Julia Gillard a previous prime minister of Australia, whose autobiography included a discussion of its underpinning principles (Gillard 2014) and the title of the article by Needham and Dickinson (2018) is a quotation from this: 'Any one of us could be among that number.' The similarity between this and the title of George's publication on unpaid care, *It Could Be You*, is striking, both underlining the precariousness of life. It follows that a system of care should engage with interdependence and vulnerability as a normal aspect of life and consider the breadth and extent of support available. A focus on social insurance schemes, for example, could ensure that the conditions within which people live are conducive to personal health and opportunities to flourish. In the post-Second World War years, that precariousness was relatively easily understood and there was political momentum to invest in social insurance.

The Australian NDIS was an example of a political decision to define a *social risk* – that is, one that carries the potential for secondary risks, and which the state recognises and accepts responsibility for addressing. As discussed in Chapter 5, Fiona Morgan has argued for care to be defined as a social risk because of the secondary risks associated with becoming an unpaid carer. The definition of social risk has traditionally been confined to contingencies against which states have already taken responsibility for protecting citizens, but Morgan (2018) argued that social risks remain even where states do not recognise them. Moreover, even where states recognise a contingency as a social risk, those affected by it might be treated differently. Unpaid care is a good example of this, because although long-term care is recognised as a social risk, it is only conceptualised as such within the public sphere. Hence those who are affected by the need for long-term care within the private, unpaid sphere remain unprotected because the family is assumed to be able to manage the risk. Like Hochschild (2003), Morgan (2018) identified the ways in which demographic and labour market changes have extended and intensified the need for long-term care, which in turn have placed pressure on the state to support unpaid care and respond to the demands of pressure groups. However, she questioned whether the action taken (in the form of the strategies and policies discussed in previous chapters) means that the state has accepted informal care as a social risk. Successive policies and strategies on unpaid care *appear* to have accepted that unpaid care is a social risk. Indeed, the Carers Strategy of 2008 acknowledged that 'everyone has the potential to become a carer and it is likely that in the future, more of us will' (HM Government 2008: 5). In Morgan's (2018) view, however, these policy actions do not amount to an acceptance of unpaid care as a social risk because they have focused on the primary risk – becoming an unpaid carer – without adequate attention to the secondary risks, such as poverty, exclusion from employment, injuries and health problems. In addition, policies do not adequately recognise the complexities of there being two risk-bearers in care relationships.

The inadequacies of the state's response to unpaid care as a social risk is evident in the inconsistencies and gaps in support, which leave unpaid carers and those they support reliant on privatised support. As a result, Morgan (2018) argued, the system of support for unpaid care generates secondary risks because of deficiencies in the care system. In addition, she pointed out that the reliance on a voluntary system of support in employment has left employees with caring responsibilities without secure rights to flexible employment, while the Carer's Allowance leaves carers exposed to the risk of poverty. As Morgan (2018) identified, while these are universal risks, in the sense that they are widespread and regularly experienced, they are not equally experienced, and the retrenchment of welfare has increased these risks and exacerbated inequalities. In the 2008 Strategy, while the state's role was accepted, the limits of its role were also clarified, while the expectation on carers was that they would have to do more. Thus, she argued, these policies have been weak, inconsistent and ineffectual and partial in their effect, leaving some needs privatised. Moreover, the care system has generated secondary risks and exacerbated problems, for example by setting the level of carers' benefits too low, leading to additional financial stresses. Inter-relational risks are also identified by Morgan (2018), which refer to the arrangements of benefits that require an unpaid carer and the person they support to decide which of them will forego financial support to enable the other to make a claim. The contentious issue of charges for services for 'substitute care' discussed in Chapter 4 can be seen in this way also.

The arguments in favour of unpaid care as a social risk cover many of the points raised in this text concerning the problematic nature of policies on unpaid care. Bearing in mind the discussion of precarity associated with a marketised system of care, the pooling of risk is a clear front-runner among the options on how to resource support for unpaid care. Following Tronto's argument (Tronto 2013) that caring systems must be 'consistent with democratic commitments to justice, equality and freedom for all', Stensöta (2020) argued that inevitably the state must be part of such care systems because unlike civil society or the market, the state has the capacity to equalise access and provision for all. She argued, further, that Tronto's fifth phase of care, 'caring with', is applicable to a publicly funded universal system in a relatively straightforward way. Stensöta reflected on the experience of Scandinavian welfare and acknowledged that a possible disadvantage of a state system is that services would become standardised rather than responsive and flexible. She emphasised, however, that her argument is for state *funding* of services, which would meet the requirement for financial security and planning to cover changes in patterns of need, not for state *provision*, which conjures up memories of institutionalised care. She also acknowledged that there might be a need for a trade-off between, on the one hand, a degree of standardisation with access for all and, on the other, flexibility and responsiveness with unequal access. As she argued, it depends on the primary policy aim. A second potential disadvantage would be that if access is based on citizenship, it would exclude non-citizens, such as asylum seekers. These potential disadvantages are capable of being tackled, however, and fundamentally, Stensöta's argument is that if the primary goal of a policy is access for all, it is necessary to consider the role of the state and to anchor care in democracy, not the market (known to be damaging) or civil society (known to be patchy in its provision) (Stensöta 2020).

Sufficiency of support is therefore a key issue, requiring more resources in the system. For Thomas (2007), an option would be for disabled people, their personal assistants and other care workers to join in common campaigning for higher value direct payments, which would enable disabled people to have control over their support without the exploitation of carers. In Thomas' suggestion there are echoes of the arguments by Parker and Clarke (2002) discussed in Chapter 5, that more services such as personal care and domestic help should be available to meet the needs of disabled people and reduce dependence on unpaid carers. A recent survey of carers, by Carers UK (2021a: 17), also identified 'having access to more personalised and better quality care for the person I care for' as a top priority for social care reform. Beckett (2007) argued that well-funded home care was needed to ensure that care tasks did not fall to family members by default. It should be organised to respect disabled people's choice and with career progression and higher status for care workers. Pickard (2012) compared the provision of care for older people by long-stay hospitals, which was free at the point of delivery, to means-tested local authority social care services and increasingly intense levels of care in families. This led her to pose the question: *why should a universal social care system not be funded out of taxation?* Thus, whether in the form of direct payments or services, a starting point for a more supportive system of social care that recognises unpaid carers would involve a major rethink of the balance between unpaid care and publicly funded services.

At the same time, having sufficient support does not satisfactorily address the question of *how* support should be provided, by whom and for whom. Like Tronto (2013), Barnes (2012) called for democratic deliberations in order to bring care thinking into political thinking. In her view, 'care full' decisions in public arenas require the participation of those who will be affected by them, recognising inequalities between people, the potential for vulnerability, and the emotional impact of being subject to social policy interventions. For Barnes (2012), such deliberative practices should take place between the private space where individual care takes place and the formal public space in which policies affecting care are made. She referred to created spaces, such as consultative events, which have the potential to be organised in 'care full' ways, in terms of how they are run and who participates. There are numerous ethical and practical questions over the provision of support for unpaid care, which call for such community spaces, where differences of perspective can be heard.

Clough (2014) considered the role of the legal system in perpetuating an atomised view of individuals and argued for the scope of analysis related to individual rights to be broadened. The need for a better reflection of interdependence is, she maintained, most starkly illustrated in the context of caring relationships, which are 'characterised by varying degrees of dependence and interdependence, reciprocal emotional needs and interwoven interests' (Clough 2014: 132). The inadequacies of law and policies are highlighted by the ethic of care, which also points the way to how these inadequacies might be addressed. Bearing in mind that relationships are not always benign, there is a strong need for an ethic of justice within care relationships, as argued by Shakespeare (2013) and Herring (2014) and discussed in Chapter 2. Like Tronto, Clough maintained that care ethics are compatible with a focus on rights but that the context of those rights must be included in the picture. In the case of people who lack mental capacity, for example, it is essential to focus on the actual position that individuals are in and whether they are capable of exercising their rights or furthering their interests. For Clough, drawing on Hankivsky (2014), the issue is not only a matter of ensuring that individual rights are upheld within care relationships but also an appreciation that rights, understood in context, can 'foster' care relationships. In practice, this perspective would introduce a basis for a formal process of negotiation and compromise in decisions affecting families and individuals. For example, Clough (2014) pointed to questions concerning decisions about the 'best interests' of people who lack mental capacity. When the rights of the disabled person are considered in isolation, decisions have the potential to overlook the impact on others who have a stake in the decision. At the same time, those others who have a stake in the decision should not be assumed to always want to make decisions in the best interests of the person who lack capacity. Clough (2014) envisaged a form of legal procedure in which such decisions are based on openness and transparency about the plurality of perspectives on decisions and the potential for conflicts of interests as well as an awareness of the family dynamics involved. Giving voice to the different parties involved would include ensuring that the interests of those who lack capacity are articulated and enable carers to set their own limits on the care they provide. These observations also reinforce Stensöta's arguments in favour of a central role for the state in care provision (Stensöta 2020) because, being based on democratic principles, the procedures that Clough (2014) and Barnes (2012) envisage would necessitate regulation and oversight.

Conclusion

In this chapter, it has been argued that there is a contradiction between the idea of care as an activity we are all involved with and the narrow perception of carers that emerged in policies since the 1990s. A focus on the widespread nature of care is a key element of the feminist ethics of care perspective, which argues that dependency and a need for care are inherent in the human condition and that an ethic of care should be in balance with an ethic of justice in caregiving and care receiving at all levels. Feminist ethicists have been subjected to critique for the limited attention they have given to justice and rights for those that receive care, although differences between contributors in the ethics of care school of thought should be taken into account, as discussed in Chapter 2. The concept of precarity, a relatively new theoretical development in gerontology, highlights how policies and practices within health and social care services have compounded the already precarious status of those who need care as well as their carers. Policies on unpaid care have not only fallen short in terms of their capacity to meet the needs of unpaid carers, therefore, but have also exacerbated these needs because of the damaging effects of the political agendas of successive governments.

Campaigns for recognition and rights by unpaid carers are an understandable response to being overlooked but have reinforced a binary division between carer and cared for. Moreover, the focus on rights for unpaid carers has not resolved the problem of inadequate resources for their support. The discussion has identified the problematic nature of paying separate attention to the needs of two individuals who are in a relationship, and it follows that an implication for policies is for better attention to the relationship between them to be the organising principle of policies and practices. A focus on relationships of care is not only a matter for professional practice with individual caring dyads. It concerns societal-level responses to human need. Tronto (2017) argued that one of the inadequacies of the neoliberal economic models is its assumption that everyone can be a self-mastering individual and this assumption can only be sustained by the location of individuals needing care within families where 'sacrifice' is the norm. Of course, the characterisation of care as sacrifice underpins the 'unsung hero' depiction of the unpaid carer, which not only runs the risk of giving offence to disabled people but also has proved to be unproductive for carers in terms of obtaining support.

Research and theorising on the care deficit has highlighted the way in which neoliberal economic models have not only devalued publicly funded provision but also shaped a perception of care in which efficiency and mechanistic delivery (*caring for*) characterises the public sphere and an idealised view of warmth and love (*caring about*) characterises the private, family sphere. In the context of a neoliberal economic system, care has thus been increasingly lacking in quantity and quality in the public sphere while in the private sphere it has continued to be taken for granted and expected to expand without limit. The effects of neoliberal economics have been experienced unequally, those with lower socioeconomic status being further disadvantaged because of their inability to purchase support in the market and because of the minimalist approach to providing publicly funded services. Unpaid care is a key part of the bigger policy agenda of cutting publicly funded welfare, as acknowledged by policy makers over the past three decades. Recognition of the universal experience of vulnerability calls for a rethink about the level of reliance on unpaid care and the impact of this on both carer and the person they support. Recognising unpaid care as a social risk is an important step towards resetting the balance of responsibility between the state and unpaid carers.

These various lines of theorising are interlinked, a fundamental acceptance of vulnerability, dependency and a need for care as basic human characteristics being an important first principle in each case. In care ethics, the centrality of care to human life undermines the drive to promote individual autonomy, independence and resilience. Butler's analysis of precarity acknowledges vulnerability as a fundamental human experience that is exacerbated by contemporary political and economic systems (Butler 2004). The concept of precarity provides a valuable explanation for the ways in which contemporary policies and practices in social care have exacerbated the marginalisation and devaluation of unpaid care, because it links these failures to wider political and economic systems rather than reducing them to professional or organisational inadequacies. A system of social care services based on the principle of social risk would provide a foundation for advancing ethically sound services that pay attention to both parties in care relationships. Tronto (2013), Barnes (2012) and Clough (2014) have all called for systems of support that are open, transparent and democratic in enabling the different interests in care relationships to be considered and for conflicts of interest to be addressed in a way that ensures care relationships promote justice for all those involved.

7

Conclusions

Introduction

In this concluding chapter, the themes that have arisen from this reflection on the history of research, policies, practices and theoretical debates on policy making and unpaid care are drawn together and the lessons to be learnt for knowledge development, policy making and practice are identified. Points to be discussed include the social status of unpaid care, the actions taken to change this through campaigning and policy action as well as the potential and limitations of policies. The role of the state in relation to unpaid care is central to this discussion. The examination of policies on unpaid care in this book has drawn attention to its marginalised status within the system of social care, reflected in the dominant perception of unpaid carers as background resources. With reference to suggested strategies for the future, the chapter includes an exploration of the potential for an ethic of justice in relationships of care, which upholds the rights of both unpaid carer and the individual who requires care and support.

As argued, many of the contemporary issues facing unpaid carers and those they support have been evident throughout decades of policy making. Over 30 years ago, the Westminster government's Social Services Committee report, discussed in Chapter 1, pointed to the need for properly costed services, including respite and specialist support, which would help carers to remain in paid employment, as well as a comprehensive system of benefits for those who give up paid employment to provide unpaid care. Over the subsequent three decades, these have been an often repeated research finding (see, for example, Banks 1999; Parker et al 2010; Pickard 2012) and are still a high priority in carers' campaigns today (Carers UK 2021a). As discussed, policies to support unpaid carers have produced important gains. For example, it was campaigning that helped to produce the Carer's Allowance, following the 1999 Carers Strategy in England. Where carers have been represented and where their voice is given due attention, unpaid care now features more strongly in policy circles. In addition, while carers must continue to campaign for more and better services for those in paid employment, the moral case for such support has been won and voluntary action by employers has benefited some carers. At the beginning of this book, three questions were posed: Why has this heavy load on unpaid care developed in a country that has a welfare system? Are carers engaged in a Sisyphean struggle to achieve their aims through government action? What has been the role and purpose of successive policies on unpaid carers and what effect have they had? A further question to be tackled in this final chapter is what are the implications of the analysis in this book for future campaigning, policy action and practice?

The potential and limitations of policies

The discussions in previous chapters have considered the various ways in which carers' interests have been taken up through the policy process. The development of local networks as well as advisory groups at national level in all four nations of the UK demonstrate the potential of effective action of groups representing unpaid carers. These have been credited with highly effective organisational and communication skills that have placed them at the heart of policy making. At the same time, unpaid care is frequently left out of relevant adjacent policy debates. For example, the White Paper on adult social care reform (DHSC 2022a) made copious references to unpaid care, while the independent report by Baroness Cavendish (DHSC 2022b) into reform of social care made few. The involvement of carers' organisations in drawing up the White Paper probably made the difference, but if recognition of carers in policy forums is reliant on the presence of their campaigning bodies, it lacks depth and authenticity.

In Chapter 5 it was argued that policies should be understood not merely as the outputs emerging from debates in political forums but as the practices that shape experiences in everyday life. Unpaid care is framed as both an unqualified good for society, enabling disabled and older people to stay out of institutions with minimal cost to the public purse *and* as a potential cost to public funds when resources for their support are called for. At the same time, carers are characterised as self-sacrificing and heroic, and their heroism is emphasised even more when the focus is on those whose role is most intense. The focus on support for unpaid carers has emphasised the need for them to be enabled to continue caring, even when conditions worsen, for the good of society. Unpaid care has been absorbed into a marketised system of social care, as was the intention in the early days of care in the community, and through the period under examination in this book there has been a continuous increase in the quantity of unpaid care provided and greater likelihood that a higher proportion of carers' time will be spent on caring. The success of policies on support for unpaid carers is therefore contingent on a wider policy agenda but as the aim of this wider agenda is to consolidate a marketised social care system with minimal state involvement, the chances of success are much reduced. And it is this wider policy agenda that should be understood *de facto* as the policy agenda on social care, and, therefore, the pre-eminent policy on unpaid carers. The impact of this wider policy agenda on carers' lives is evident in their continuing struggle to cope with fewer publicly funded services. The policies listed in Table 3.1 have played a role in softening this impact for some carers but are designed to operate within this wider policy agenda and not to challenge it. The reshaping of social care over the past three decades has also included an increase in activity by the voluntary sector, including carers' organisations, in service provision. This, too, has reinforced the drive to efficiency because the voluntary sector organisations offer cheaper services than those run by the state. In addition, while the social care system benefits from the involvement of voluntary organisations' expertise by experience, it is inherently exploitative, and the exploitation of voluntary organisations mirrors the exploitation of unpaid carers.

There are fundamental tensions within the policy agenda on unpaid care and these result in, at best, patchy and uneven practices. Policies to relieve the stress faced by unpaid carers are undermined by the impact of cuts to services for disabled children and adults as well as older people and the relief of unpaid carers' stress will always be measured against the savings that their contribution represents for the social care system. Assumptions about the likely pressures on social care arising from an ageing population have been a major factor in the priority given to cost-cutting. Indeed, demographic trends have been a driver of policies for decades. Underlying this, however, has been the political strategy to change the nature of the welfare state in the UK. This political agenda, together with the framing of care within the family as a superior option to institutionalised care, produced what Parker and Clarke (2002) described as the 'unholy trio' of policies: low cost services; idealised family care; and non-institutional support. This is to the disadvantage of unpaid carers in general, with more disadvantages for those with fewer resources. The years of austerity since 2010 have reinforced already established trends towards greater social inequalities and these have been reflected in unequal access to services and injustices within the system, in which those with fewest resources are hit hardest by austerity's effects. The impact on carers has, as discussed, been immense and the growing crisis in the cost of living at the time of writing will exacerbate an already critical situation.

Reflections on rights, recognition and resources

Over three decades the rights of unpaid carers have increased in the following main respects: their right to an assessment of needs on equal terms with those of service users; the right of some carers in paid employment to request flexible working arrangements; and the right of some to carers' benefits. In addition, carers who are in paid employment have associative rights under the Equality Act, 2010 and, as discussed previously, are campaigning to strengthen this by having caring declared the tenth protected characteristic under the Equality Act, 2010. The evidence discussed in this text demonstrates that the rights carers have already gained are not being recognised in practice, which raises a question about the value of this campaign. Moreover, age and disability are already protected characteristics under the Equality Act, 2010 and evidence of the outcomes of this protection on older and disabled people has not been encouraging. Rights are eclipsed by political priorities and, as discussed, carers' right to flexible working conditions cannot be exercised when alternative forms of care have closed down. As argued, caring is by its nature an interpersonal matter (Milne 2020). Rights associated with the assessment of needs, flexible working conditions or attention from health professionals make sense only in terms of there being another person in the picture. This is not to suggest that a focus on rights is futile, because carers can benefit from the protections of human rights legislation, as the Northern Ireland Human Rights Commission (NIHRC 2014) argued, but to point out its limitations. While the need for better recognition of carers is undeniable, there remains a question over whether the best way to achieve this is through a pursuit of specific rights for carers.

In some ways, the carer identity has proved cumbersome, especially as increasingly it has become a prerequisite for access to services, which places additional responsibility on carers for obtaining support. This is, arguably, the opposite of recognition as envisaged, in which what carers *do* rather than what they *are* would be seen and acknowledged by those with the authority to give them support. The emphasis placed on encouraging unpaid carers to come forward and identify themselves as carers to gain access to services draws attention to the dual framing of carers in policies discussed in Chapter 6. Carers are at one and the same time considered to be a diverse and widespread group *and* a specific category eligible to access support and services. These different perspectives align with the perceptions identified by Twigg and Atkin (1994), discussed in Chapter 4. When carers are characterised as co-workers, their contribution is highly valued. When it comes to providing resources for their support, their identity as co-clients narrows to limit the numbers who are eligible. Even those who are eligible have experienced difficulties in obtaining access to services, as identified by Rand and Malley (2014) with waiting lists operating and inaccurate information acting as forms of rationing. In policy debates, there has been a tendency to highlight the worst case as a way of framing unpaid carers. As discussed in Chapter 1, the House of Commons Social Services Committee (House of Commons 1990) emphasised that they were interested in those carers with burdens that were impossible to exaggerate. Over the decades since then, restrictions on resources have meant that local authorities must focus on those in greatest need and the definition of greatest need has become harsher as the effects of austerity have strengthened. As discussed in

Chapter 5, this was evident in the Older Carers project, when it emerged that the carers' organisation contracted to conduct carers' assessments had, itself, taken on responsibility for ensuring their focus was on carers 'on the cusp of collapse' (O'Rourke 2021).

A historical perspective clarifies how the idea that publicly funded support must be reserved for those who are in dire straits has become normalised and entrenched within the system of social care. In addition, the concept of 'unmet need' has become part of the everyday language of social care practice, which speaks volumes about the normalisation of neglect. An unmet need (as opposed to a need) is a need that has been identified as requiring attention but not given any. As a result of this very unpromising context, it becomes difficult to envisage a policy to support unpaid carers. The success of carers' campaigns in establishing the moral case of all carers to be recognised and supported falls foul of the wider social care policy that focuses on those in greatest need. With the benefit of a historical perspective, it can be argued that there has never been a policy decision about what would be a fair deal for carers. Instead, policies focus on enabling carers to cope, thus already assuming a negative starting point. Even in supportive strategies that included extra funding, such as the Carers Strategy of 2008, the purpose of the policy was spelt out in the introduction which referred to carers' 'increasingly vital role' in managing the growing demands on the care system and on carers. The strategy was to help carers to face 'everyday challenges and obstacles' and to provide respite (HM Government 2008: 2). Acknowledgement by policy makers that the strain on carers is unbearable has become part of the framing of unpaid care and its place in the social care system. Arguably, the focus on recognition has brought carers out of the background to the foreground but has not stopped them from being seen as resources.

There was a change towards a broader definition of carers in the 2014 legislation in England and Wales, which led to changes in practice but whether these were to the carers' benefit is arguable. Fernandez et al (2021) commented that carers' position as co-clients was consolidated in the 2014 Care Act in England, because the requirement on local authorities to ensure that carers were offered an assessment where there is an appearance of need placed carers on a par with service users. This was hailed at the time by carers' organisations and their supporters as a success, but local authority managers were deeply concerned about the unknown numbers of additional assessments that would be requested. This focused their minds on ways of managing what might otherwise be an unmanageable challenge, given their crisis-level resources. Different strategies were introduced in practice, as discussed in Chapter 4, including more contracting out of assessments; introducing a two-stage process of assessment, less in-depth at the first stage; broadening the base of practitioners qualified to conduct assessments; and managing longer waiting lists for assessments. According to Fernandez et al (2021), in England the expected increase in assessments did not emerge. Instead, there was a continuation of the long-standing decline in the number of assessments conducted. Statutory interventions to support carers have been increasingly confined to situations where the carers' needs are 'complex', as flagged up by the initial assessment. Significantly, then, it is the relationship between the needs of the carer and the person they care for that produces the kind of complex circumstances that stimulate higher level intervention.

The Care Act, 2014 in England and the Social Services and Well-being (Wales) Act, 2014 bear all the hallmarks of the contradictory perceptions in policies between, on one hand, carers as co-workers (rather than an 'appendage' or 'mere co-client') and on the other hand carers as co-clients (with equal rights to an assessment of needs). This contradiction has endured since the beginning of policy making to support unpaid carers. The Carers (Scotland) Act 2016 also adopted a broader view of carers and entitled them to an adult carers support plan (similar to an assessment) if there was an appearance of need. It was based on a stronger perception of unpaid carers as co-workers, which had been building since 2000. At the same time, if the assessment identified a need for services, calculations of the carers' eligibility for these placed them squarely in the co-client category. In all three countries, the implementation of this legislation has proven somewhat disappointing. The preventive work that was envisaged, through bolstering the wellbeing of carers in general, has been curtailed through lack of resources and the loss of regular services for people who are supported by unpaid carers has led to a reduction in regular breaks and respite as well as difficulties for carers in accessing or remaining in paid work. The role of the market as provider of alternative services has not been beneficial in general, but, as Pollock et al (2021) identified in relation to care of people with dementia, benefits have been confined to those who have the means to pay the high charges they impose. In addition, the logic of the market has been to emphasise efficiency so that even where unpaid carers are able to take a break, the service is not always beneficial to the service user.

A broad and inclusive definition of unpaid carers has great merit, given the weight of evidence that shows the diverse and widespread nature of unpaid care. This definition also points to the need for preventive policies and practices that can benefit more carers and lift professional practice out of the reactive, 'fire-fighting' mode that is inevitable when attention is on those on the cusp of collapse. Austerity budgets over the past decade have stood in the way of previously common forms of support for carers, such as regular direct payments, which were often awarded with relatively little fuss, to enable carers to take time out in ways that suited them. This was recognition of the importance of time off, and potentially highly beneficial, if direct payments were sufficiently generous to allow for satisfactory replacement care arrangements. A broad and inclusive definition of unpaid care also supports the whole family approach to assessments, which has featured in England and Wales since 2014, to a greater or lesser extent. In Wales, the continuing practice of joint assessment of needs is intended to promote attention to both service user and carer at the same time, which would be a promising approach if resources were sufficient to provide services to meet the assessed needs. The whole family approach in the Care Act 2014 in England was present in the policy and guidance but was lost in the implementation, as priority was given to the separation of assessments within a more fragmented system. A whole family approach to needs assessments would focus attention on a wider set of needs and potential sources of support but would require skilled practice in assessment, not a formulaic approach, and willingness on the part of professionals to engage with the issues and challenges involved in unpaid care and to acknowledge the inextricable links between service users, unpaid carers and paid care workers in developing a whole family approach.

The perception of unpaid care as both something we all do and something that concerns a specific group appears inherently inconsistent. When considered in the context of the life course, however, the apparent inconsistency can be reconciled. The analysis by Katz (2020), discussed in Chapter 6, examined how dependency and vulnerability can be understood as a human characteristic that is experienced differently through the life course. It follows that unpaid care can be understood in a similar way. It is both something that concerns us all but also something of particular concern to specific individuals at any one time. This points to the need for policies that are focused on making access to support easier for individuals at the time they need it. It does not require a gigantic leap of imagination to envisage, for example, ease of access to advice and information, flexible working arrangements and adequate benefits that are made available when caring responsibilities increase. These are the kinds of support that have already been itemised in successive strategies for carers. To make them a reality would require a change in the political agenda and an acceptance that there is a cost to caring, currently borne by those who are in an unpaid care relationship, many of whom feel their willingness to do it has been taken for granted. It is an obvious point, perhaps, but to suggest that support for carers would be satisfactory if only adequate resources were made available is to view the problem from the wrong end. It is, rather, that under the current political and economic regime, the level of resources is set at a level that *guarantees* that unpaid care will never have sufficient resources. Despite the success of unpaid carers in voicing their demands in policy-making circles, they have not yet succeeded in achieving recognition within policies, that is, in Sayer's terms, backed up by equality of treatment, resources and opportunities (Sayer 2011).

The marginalisation of unpaid care in practice

A similar problem arises in relation to practice also. The continuing assumptions made by front-line practitioners about unpaid carers as background resources were discussed in Chapter 4. Reflecting on this discussion, it can be argued that although carers continue to be background resources, they are less invisible now than when Twigg and Atkin (1994) developed their model. Unpaid care is now factored into service planning and provision in local authorities. Organisations representing unpaid carers occupy a role as partners in many places. Arguably, it is still largely perceived as a specialist interest, however, rather than being of central importance to social work and social care services in general. This marginalisation is reflected also in publications and in research agendas, where unpaid care is generally considered a specialist sphere of interest. Publications on social work and social care still routinely make scant reference, if any, to unpaid care, as Barnes (2012) also commented. Instead, service users are characterised as somewhat isolated individuals and the focus on professional practice often misses the social relationships of service users. For example, drawing on the work of Tronto (2010), Hudson (2021) presented a discussion of ethics in social work practice and argued that Tronto's model of an ethic of care applies to front-line practitioners, politicians, policy makers, managers and owners of private companies. He developed an argument about ethical commissioning practices to make a series of very valuable suggestions. He also acknowledged (albeit briefly) that unpaid carers bear the brunt of diminished access to support services in the context of austerity. Somehow, however, the key point of Tronto's argument about the centrality of care to human life was missing from his analysis. This is not unusual, and it is concerning that commentators in social work and social policy incorporate unpaid care into their analyses so infrequently.

Hudson (2021) also expressed regret over the low numbers of carers' assessments since the Care Act, 2014 in England. Certainly, as discussed in Chapter 4, front-line practitioners' lack of enthusiasm for conducting carers assessments can be explained in part by the lack of services available, which calls into question the point of an assessment, but it must be acknowledged also that the marginalised position of unpaid carers in social work and social policy texts is also a contributing factor. It is little wonder that professionals have difficulty envisaging a different approach to practice when unpaid care is in such a marginal position. As Mitchell et al (2014) pointed out at that time, social workers had difficulty imagining how carers' envisaged outcomes could fit in to the system of social care. Now, after further years of austerity and financial crisis, they are even less likely to be able to do so. Enabling this to happen requires a more fundamental shift of emphasis in the framework of practice as well as in professional conduct. Unpaid care is, as is often stated in policy documents, the largest sphere of practice in the entire social care system, yet it is a minor element in debates about the future of social care. Changes cannot be imposed on existing patterns of practice but require a more fundamental rethink about the role and potential of professional social workers and care managers. The discussion in Chapter 6 suggests that the task of changing attitudes towards practice with carers requires more than an assertion of carers' rights, especially when professional ethics have been more focused on service users' rights. Bringing unpaid care out of the background would, in Tronto's terms, require attentiveness on the part of professionals to those who provide care as well as those who need it, because those who need it are not isolated individuals but connected to others (Tronto 1993). Arksey et al identified the ability to adjust to and manage change as one of carers' desired outcomes of the support received from service providers (Arksey et al 2007). This is arguably a task that professional social workers are well able to take on, because enabling people to manage change is a core professional skill. Another desired outcome was being able to control the amount of support they provide. Enabling individuals to adjust to change also involves assisting unpaid carers in deciding how much adjustment they want to make and ensuring that they have a choice. Facilitating choice for carers inevitably involves finding alternative sources of support. At present, the cost of replacement care falls to the service user in all four countries of the UK, which draws attention to the potential for conflicts of interest between the carer and the person they care for, as discussed. Facing these challenging circumstances would certainly require high levels of competence and skill but, again, are well suited to the role of professional social workers and, with the right resources, the whole family approach offers a promising framework.

The argument returns over and over again to the issue of resources, and without sufficient resources it will not be possible to make the changes needed to improve the circumstances of unpaid care. Importantly, these resources are necessary to ensure that the care provided will enhance the lives of service users and their carers, not only to enable carers to pursue paid employment or other activities in life beyond caring. In addition, while sufficient resources are necessary, they are not the complete answer because a change in perspective on unpaid care is also required in practice, to overcome its marginalised position.

Challenges for the wider policy context

This discussion of policy and practice leads to a concluding argument concerning the role of the state in funding, providing and regulating care and determining the conditions of unpaid care. As discussed in Chapter 1, in the 1990s state-run services were under fire as institutionalised, inefficient, poor quality and oppressive to disabled and older people. Alternative forms of provision through unpaid care as well as the voluntary sector and private, for-profit sectors were easily presented in more favourable terms when care in the community was introduced. A critique of the wider political agenda on care, however, draws attention to the ideology involved, which promotes individual self-reliance and consumer acumen as well as marketised arrangements for service provision with a corresponding reduction in the size and importance of the state. Indeed, the emphasis on a reduction in state involvement in care provision is bound up with the characterisation of the ideal self-reliant citizen. In Chapter 6, the ideology of self-reliance was challenged and alternative ideas presented, related to human dependency and the centrality of care. A broader perspective on care as something we are all involved in creates a different perspective on dependency, which is no longer associated with a category of people who are dependants but is a characteristic shared in common. This broader perspective also requires greater recognition of the complexity of care relationships, including the potential for abuse of power as well as the potential for great satisfaction. The broader perspective is consistent with many of the campaigning aims of organisations of carers as well as those of older and disabled people.

Recent theorising in gerontology that draws on the concept of precarity also advances understanding of vulnerability in human life, through a focus on the additional vulnerabilities faced by older people within care systems. The marketised system of social care has introduced new forms of vulnerability and insecurity, related to the unravelling of the welfare system. The increase in unpaid care also poses risks for both carer and the person they care for, especially when there is inadequate support, inadequate understanding of care needs and fewer breaks for carers, as discussed in Chapter 4. At the same time, given its oppressive history, it is not surprising that there is hesitation about an expanded role for the state. The evidence is plain that state services can be abusive in their exercise of power over service users as well as neglectful of their needs. Two counter-arguments can be considered: first, evidence also shows that voluntary and private sectors can also be institutionalising and abusive and, second, a larger role for the state does not necessarily mean a return to institutions, or even necessarily a larger role in service provision. The argument here is about the responsibility of the state to ensure that needs are met. This could be by a range of independent organisations and community groups as well as through unpaid care.

The focus on care as something we all need and are involved in also points to the potential for a universal system of support in social care, capable of reaching many different levels of need and maximising the preventive capacity of care. As Stensöta (2020) has argued, only the state has the capacity to ensure care for all, because markets produce unequal outcomes, depending on the profitability of services, while voluntary organisations (or civic society) operate where they have the resources to do so. Indeed, the economic crisis current at the time of writing shows in stark relief the increased likelihood of service provider failure in all sectors. Unless the state ensures that services are provided where they are needed, then unpaid carers will continue to pick up responsibility. As discussed in Chapter 6, a social risk approach has much to recommend it, especially as this would correspond with the argument concerning the life-course understanding of dependency and likelihood of being a carer. Morgan (2018) argued that unpaid care qualifies on all fronts as a social risk, including the evidence of secondary risks arising from the experience of being an unpaid carer. Research on the impact on carers of their caring role, discussed in Chapter 2, stretches back over three decades, and as argued by Henwood et al (2019), this has identified more about the negatives than the positives of unpaid care and little unequivocal evidence of the benefits of professional interventions. These secondary risks make unpaid care a prime candidate for recognition as a social risk – that being a risk that the state should take responsibility for, based on the principle of collective provision. This is not to hark back to an imaginary golden period of the welfare state, but to recognise the value of the principle of shared risk in the context of social care in the 21st century. Accepting that unpaid care is a risk shared by everyone, it follows that the resources to fund it should be collectively organised.

The shortcomings of the present system of social care and of the political and economic policy context that shape it are clear, as the discussion of the care deficit in Chapter 6 highlighted. This still leaves the question of how provision should be organised and funded, however, and what role unpaid care should occupy within this newly organised system. Where should responsibility lie and to what extent should a relationship based on family ties be considered a basis for care provision? The findings of researchers over the entire period discussed in this text has led to the conclusion that the balance between paid and unpaid care requires recalibration (see Parker and Clarke 2002; Beckett 2007; Thomas 2007; Morgan 2018). As already argued, these decisions should include individual choice about whether to provide unpaid care at all and, if so, how much, as well as choice for an individual about how they wish to be supported. As discussed in Chapter 6, both Tronto (2013) and Barnes (2012) have called for democratic deliberations in which care can be brought into political debate and thinking. Tronto made the pertinent point that the aim of such deliberations is not to establish a standard picture of what constitutes a fair amount of unpaid care but to establish a fair basis upon which such decisions can be made.

There is, as Clough (2014) and Shakespeare (2013) argued, a need for an ethic of justice in care relationships. There are many examples of injustice in care settings, not only in those that are directly abusive but also in those that deny service users choice and subject them to routinised services. But injustices in care are often framed as 'poor care' and access to justice is routinely denied to individuals within the care system. Addressing this failure is not only about ensuring *access* to justice, however, it is also preventive, being about ensuring that within the system there are measures in place to ensure that power relations within a care relationship do not become abusive. As Clough (2014) expressed it, the need is to ensure that rights are upheld in ways that *foster* care relationships. In this endeavour, it is the relationship that matters most and the perspectives of both (or all) parties need to be given fair consideration, based on recognition of equal worth. The diversity of unpaid care relationships points to the plurality of perspectives on how they should be supported and demands that decisions are made in an open and transparent way. Reflecting on Dilnot's words, the primary task is to bring social care out of the shadows and to acknowledge that the need for care and to care is a social risk. Acknowledgement of this could result in more fruitful lines of campaigning and more coherent policies.

References

ACAS (2012) *Code of Practice on Employment of Carers*. London: Advisory, Conciliation and Arbitration Service.

ADSS (Association of Directors of Social Services) (2001) *The Carers and Disabled Children Act 2000 Policy and Practice Guidance: Response of the Association of Directors of Social Services*. London: ADSS.

Alcock, P. (2010) Building the Big Society: A new policy environment for the third sector in England. In H. Kippen, G. Stoker and S. Griffiths (eds) *Public Services: A New Reform Agenda*. London: Bloomsbury.

Allen, C. (1998) The care programme approach: The experiences and views of carers. *Mental Health Care*, 1(5), 160–162.

Andrews, R. and Martin, S. (2010) Regional variations in public service outcomes: The impact of policy divergence in England, Scotland and Wales. *Regional Studies*, 44(8), 919–934.

Anfilogoff, T. (2018) Weathering the perfect storm: Facing the challenge of maintaining gains for carers against a background of shrinking resources in one area of England. *International Journal of Care and Caring*, 2(1), 125–132.

Arber, S. and Gilbert, N. (1989) Men: The forgotten carers. *Sociology*, 23(1), 111–118.

Arber, S. and Ginn, J. (1990) The meaning of informal care: Gender and the contribution of elderly people. *Ageing & Society*, 10(4), 429–454.

Arber, S. and Ginn, J. (1992) Class and caring: A forgotten dimension. *Sociology*, 26(4), 619–634.

Arksey, H. and Glendinning, C. (2007) Choice in the context of informal care-giving. *Health and Social Care in the Community*, **15**(2), 165–175.

Arksey, H., Hepworth, D. and Qureshi, H. (2000) *Carers' Needs and the Carers Act: An Evaluation of the Process and Outcomes of Assessment*. York: Social Policy Research Unit, University of York.

Arksey, H., O'Malley, L., Baldwin, S., Harris, J., Mason, A. and Golder, S. (2002) Literature review report: Services to support carers of people with mental health problems. York: University of York.

Arksey, H., Jackson, K., Wallace, A., Baldwin, S., Golder, S., Newbronner, E. and Hare, P. (2003) *Access to Health Care for Carers: Barriers and Interventions*. Report for the National Co-ordinating Centre for NHS Service Delivery and Organisation R&D. York: University of York.

Arksey, H., Beresford, B., Glendinning, C., Greco, V. and Sloper, T. (2007) Outcomes for parents with disabled children and carers of disabled or older adults: Similarities, differences and the implications for assessment practice. York: University of York, 1–22.

Armstrong, P. and Armstrong, H. (2020) *The Privatization of Care: The Case of Nursing Homes*. New York: Routledge.

References

Ash, A. (2014) *Safeguarding Older People from Abuse: Critical Contexts to Policy and Practice*. Bristol: Policy Press.

Asthana, A. (2017) Take care of your elderly mothers and fathers, says Tory minister. *The Guardian*, 31 January.

Atkins, G., Dalton, G., Phillips, A. and Stojanivic, A. (2021) *Devolved Public Services: The NHS, Schools and Social Care in the Four Nations*. London: Institute for Government.

Ayres, S. and Marsh, A. (2014) Reflections on contemporary debates in policy studies. *Policy and Politics*, 41(4), 643–663.

Azong, J.A. and Wilińska, M. (2017) Into a footnote: Unpaid care work and the Equality Budget in Scotland. *European Journal of Women's Studies*, 24(3), 218–232.

Baldwin, S. and Twigg, J. (1991) Women and community care: Reflections on a debate. In M. Maclean and D. Groves (eds) *Women's Issues in Social Policy*. London: Routledge, pp 117–135.

Banks, P. (1999) *Carer support: Time for a change of direction?* Policy Discussion Paper. London: King's Fund.

Banks, P. and Cheeseman, C. (1999) *Taking Action to Support Carers: A Carers Impact Guide for Commissioners and Managers*. London: King's Fund.

Barclay, P.M. (1982) *Social Workers: Their Role and Tasks*. London: National Institute for Social Work.

Barnes, C. and Mercer, G. (2003) *Disability*. Cambridge: Polity.

Barnes, M. (2006) *Caring and Social Justice*. Basingstoke: Palgrave Macmillan.

Barnes, M. (2012) *Care in Everyday Life: An Ethic of Care in Practice*. Bristol: Policy Press.

Beckett, C. (2007) Women, disability and care: Good neighbours or uneasy bedfellows. *Critical Social Policy*, 27(3), 360–380.

Berzins, K.M. and Atkinson, J.M. (2009) Service users' and carers' views of the Named Person provisions under the Mental Health (Care and Treatment) (Scotland) Act 2003. *Journal of Mental Health*, 18(3), 207–215.

Betts, J. and Thompson, J. (2016) Carers: Legislation, policy and practice. Paper 24/17, Northern Ireland Assembly NIAR 43-17.

Biziewska, D. and Palattiyil, G. (2022) Promoting human rights or increasing expectations? Effects of Self-Directed Support on the realisation of human rights in Scotland. *Disability & Society*, 1–21.

Bottery, S. (2021) *The Social Care White Paper: Not Wrong, Just Not Moving Far Enough in the Right Direction*. London: King's Fund.

Boushel, M. (2000) What kind of people are we? 'Race', anti-racism and social welfare research. *British Journal of Social Work*, 30(1), 71–89.

Bowes, A. and Bell, D. (2007) Free personal care for older people in Scotland: Issues and implications. *Social Policy and Society*, 6(3), 435–445.

Brannelly, T. and Barnes, M. (2022) *Researching with Care: Applying Feminist Care Ethics to Research Practice*. Bristol: Policy Press.

Brimblecombe, N., Pickard, L., King, D. and Knapp, M. (2018) Barriers to receipt of social care services for working carers and the people they care for in times of austerity. *Journal of Social Policy*, 47(2), 215–233.

Buckner, L. and Yeandle, S. (2007) *Valuing Carers: Calculating the Value of Carers' Support*. London: Carers UK.

Buckner, L. and Yeandle, S. (2015) *Valuing Carers 2015: The Rising Value of Carers' Support*. London: Carers UK.

Burchardt, T., Obolenskaya, P. and Vizard, P. (2016) Adult social care. In R Lupton, T. Burchardt, J. Hills, K. Stewart and P. Vizard (eds) *Social Policy in a Cold Climate*. Bristol: Policy Press, pp 187– 214.

Butler, J. (2004) *Precarious Life: The Powers of Mourning and Violence*. London: Verso.

Butler, P. (2013) Jeremy Hunt: UK should adopt Asian culture of caring for the elderly. *The Guardian*, 18 October.

Bytheway, B. and Johnson, J. (1998) The social construction of 'carers'. In A. Symonds and A. Kelly (eds) *The Social Construction of Community Care*. Basingstoke: Macmillan, pp 241–253.

Cameron, A. and Lart, R. (2003) Factors promoting and obstacles hindering joint working: A systematic review of the research evidence. *Journal of Integrated Care*, 11(2), 9–17.

Cameron, A., Lart, R., Bostock, L. and Coomber, C. (2014) Factors that promote and hinder joint and integrated working between health and social care services: A review of research literature. *Health & Social Care in the Community*, 22(3), 225–233.

Campbell-Smith, D. (2008) *Follow the Money: The Audit Commission, Public Money and the Management of Public Services 1983–2008*. London: Allen Lane.

Care 21 (2006) *The Future of Unpaid Care in Scotland: Headline Report and Recommendations*. Edinburgh: Scottish Executive.

Care and Social Services Inspectorate Wales (2017) Carers engagement overview report. WG31783. Welsh Government.

Carers National Association (1997) In on the Act? Social Services' Experience of the First Year of the Carers Act. London: Carers National Association

Carers Northern Ireland (2013) *Response to Transforming Your Care: Vision to Action*. Consultation Response January 2013. Belfast: Carers Northern Ireland.

Carers Northern Ireland (2021) *State of Caring 2021 in Northern Ireland*. Belfast: Carers Northern Ireland.

Carers Trust (2020) *Our Impact Report: Year Ended 31 March 2020*. Hornchurch: Carers Trust.

Carers Trust (2022) Homepage. Available at: www.carers.org

Carers Trust Wales (2022) *Carer Aware Project*. Carers Trust Wales. Available at: http://carers.org/carer-aware-project

Carers UK (2012a) *Sandwich Caring: Combining Childcare with Caring for Older or Disabled Relatives*. London: Carers UK.

Carers UK (2012b) *Growing the Care Market: Turning a Demographic Challenge into and Economic Opportunity*. London: Carers UK.

Carers UK (2014) *Caring and Family Finances Inquiry UK Report*. London: Carers UK.

Carers UK (2015) *The Care Act 2014 and Carers: Opportunities for Change Research and Practice Briefing*. March. London: Carers UK.

Carers UK (2018) Submission to the House of Lords Economic Affairs Committee Inquiry into Social Care Funding in England. Evidence submission. October. London: Carers UK.

Carers UK (2019a) Women's Budget Group Commission on a Gender-Equal Economy: Examples of transformative policies and practices. Evidence submission. London: Carers UK.

Carers UK (2019b) Opposition Day Debate Briefing for MPs: Carers and the social care system. London: Carers UK.

Carers UK (2020) Caring behind closed doors: Six months on. The continued impact of the Coronavirus (COVID-19) pandemic on unpaid care. London: Carers UK.

Carers UK (2021) *State of Caring 2021: A Snapshot of Unpaid Care in the UK*. London: Carers UK.

Carers UK (2022a) *Policy Briefing on Adult Social Care White Paper: People at the Heart of Care*. London: Carers UK.

Carers UK (2022b) *Under Pressure: Carers and the Cost of Living Crisis*. London: Carers UK.

Carers Wales (2018) Health and Social Care Committee: Inquiry into the impact of the Social Services Wellbeing (Wales) Act 2014 in relation to carers. Inquiry response, September. Cardiff: Carers UK Wales.

Carlisle, C. (2000) The search for meaning in HIV and AIDS: The carers' experience. *Qualitative Health Research*, 10(6), 750–765.

Carpenter, J. and Sbarini, S. (1996) Involving service users and carers in the care programme approach. *Journal of Mental Health*, 5(5), 483–488.

Carpenter, J., Schneider, J., McNiven, F., Brandon, T., Stevens, R. and Wooff, D. (2004) Integration and targeting of community care for people with severe and enduring mental health problems: Users' experiences of the care programme approach and care management. *British Journal of Social Work*, 34(3), 313–333.

Clements, L. (2016) *Carers and their Rights: England*. 6th edition. London: Carers UK.

Clements, L., Bangs, J. and Holzhausen, E. (2008) *Individual Budgets and Carers*. Available at: www.lukeclements.co.uk

Clements, L., Bangs, J. and Holzhausen, E. (2009) Individual budgets and carers. Updated briefing paper. Available at: www.lukeclements.co.uk

Clements, L., Holzhausen, E. and Bangs, J. (2011) *The Equality Act 2010 and Carers*. Available at: www.lukeclements.co.uk

Clough, B. (2014) What about us? A case for legal recognition of interdependence in informal care relationships. *Journal of Social Welfare and Family Law*, 36(2), 129–148.

Colebatch, H. and Hoppe, R. (2018) Introduction to the handbook on policy, process and governing. In H. Colebatch and R. Hoppe (eds) *Handbook on Policy, Process and Governing*. Cheltenham: Edward Elgar, pp 1–12.

Colebatch, H., Hoppe, R. and Noordegraaf, M. (2010) The lessons for policy work. In H. Colebatch, R. Hoppe and M. Noordegraaf (eds) *Working for Policy*. Amsterdam: Amsterdam University Press, pp 227–245.

Coles, B. (2015) A 'suitable person': An 'insider' perspective. *British Journal of Learning Disabilities*, 43(2), 135–141.

Cook, T. (2007) *The History of the Carers' Movement*. London: Carers UK.

Cooper, C., Selwood, A. and Livingston, G. (2008) The prevalence of elder abuse and neglect: A systematic review. *Age and Ageing*, 3(7), 151–160.

Cramer, H. and Carlin, J. (2008) Family-based short breaks (respite) for disabled children: Results from the fourth national survey. *British Journal of Social Work*, 38(6), 1060–1075.

Crowley, K., Stewart, J., Kay, A. and Head, B.W. (2020) *Reconsidering Policy: Complexity, Governance and the State*. Bristol: Policy Press.

D'Rosario, M. and Lloyd-Cape, M. (2021) False economy: The economic benefits of the NDIS and the consequences of government cost-cutting. Report, Per Capita. Available at: www.percapita.org.au

Dahlberg, L., Demack, S. and Bambra, C. (2007) Age and gender of informal carers: A population-based study in the UK. *Health & Social Care in the Community*, 15(5), 439–445.

Dalley, G. (1983) Ideologies of care: A feminist contribution to the debate. *Critical Social Policy*, 3(8), 72–81.

Davies, J.S. and Thompson, E. (2016) Austerity realism and the governance of Leicester. In M. Bevir and R.A.W. Rhodes (eds) *Rethinking Governance: Ruling, Rationalities and Resistance*. London: Routledge, pp 144–161.

Dayan, M. and Heenan, D. (2019) *Change or Collapse: Lessons from the Drive to Reform Health and Social Care in Northern Ireland*. London: Nuffield Trust.

Del Bono, E., Sala, E. and Hancock, R. (2009) Older carers in the UK: Are there really gender differences? New analysis of the Individual Sample of Anonymised Records from the 2001 UK Census. *Health & Social Care in the Community*, 17(3), 267–273.

Department of Health, Social Services and Public Safety/An Roinn Sláinte Seirbhísí Sóisialta agus Sábháilteachta Poiblí (2005) *Carers and Direct Payments Act (Northern Ireland) 2002: Carers' Assessment and Information Guidance*. Belfast: Department of Health, Social Services and Public Safety/An Roinn Sláinte Seirbhísí Sóisialta agus Sábháilteachta Poiblí.

References

DH (Department of Health) (1989) *Caring for People: Community Care in the Next Decade and Beyond.* London: HMSO.

DH (1990) *Community Care in the Next Decade and Beyond: Policy Guidance.* London: HMSO.

DH (1991) *Caring for People: Getting it Right for Carers.* London: Stationery Office Books.

DH (1995) *Carers (Recognition and Services) Act 1995.* London: DH.

DH (1996) *Carers (Recognition and Services) Act 1995: Policy Guidance and Practice Guide.* London: DH.

DH (1999b) *National Service Framework for Mental Health.* London: DH.

DH (2001a) *Carers and Disabled Children Act 2000. Carers and People with Parental Responsibility for Disabled Children: Practice Guidance.* London: D

DH (2001b) *Valuing People: A New Strategy for Learning Disability for the 21st Century.* Cm5086. London: DH.

DH (2007) *Putting People First: A Shared Vision and Commitment to the Transformation of Adult Social Care.* London: DH.

DH (2014) *Fact Sheet 8: The Care Act – the Law for Carers.* London: DH.

DHSC (Department of Health and Social Care) (2018) *Carers Action Plan 2018–2020, Supporting Carers Today: One Year on Progress Review.* London: Department of Health and Social Care.

DHSC (2022a) *People at the Heart of Care: Adult Social Care Reform White Paper.* London: Department of Health and Social Care

DHSC (2022b) *Social Care: Independent Report by Baroness Cavendish.* London: DHSC.

DHSS (Department of Health and Social Security) (1981) *Growing Older.* London: HMSO

DHSS (Department of Health and Social Services) (1991) *People First: Community Care in Northern Ireland for the 1990s.* Belfast: DHSS.

DHSSPS (Department of Health, Social Services and Public Safety) (2002) *Valuing Carers: A Strategy for Carers in Northern Ireland.* Belfast: DHSSPS.

Dickinson, H. and Kavanagh, A. (2022) With a return to Labor government, it's time for an NDIS 'reset'. *The Conversation.* Available at: https://theconversation.com/with-a-return-to-labor-government-its-time-for-an-ndis-reset-183628

Dilnot, A. (2011) *Fairer Care Funding: The Report of the Commission on Funding of Care and Support.* London: The Stationery Office.

Dilnot, A. (2022) Jeremy hunt put vital social care reforms on hold: A failed Britain's most vulnerable people. *The Guardian,* 17 November.

Donoghue, M. and Edmiston, D. (2020) Gritty citizens? Exploring the logic and limits of resilience in UK social policy during times of socio-material insecurity. *Critical Social Policy,* 40(1), 7–29.

Doran, T., Drever, F. and Whitehead, M. (2003) Health of young and elderly informal carers: Analysis of UK census data. *BMJ,* 327(7428), 1388.

Drakeford, M. (2012) Wales in the age of austerity. *Critical Social Policy*, 32(3), 454–466.

DWP (Department for Work and Pensions) (2021) *Family Resources Survey: Financial Year 2019–2020*. London: DWP.

Easton, D. (1965) *A Systems Analysis of Political Life*. New York: Wiley.

Eckersley, P. and Tobin, P. (2019) The impact of austerity on policy capacity in local government. *Policy & Politics*, 47(3), 455–472.

Exley, S. (2021) Open policy making in the UK: To whom might policy formulation be 'opening up'? *Journal of Social Policy*, 50(3), 451–469.

Farnsworth, K. (2021) Retrenched, reconfigured and broken: The British welfare state after a decade of austerity. *Social Policy and Society*, 20(1), 77–96.

Fernandez, J.-L., Marczak, J., Snell, T., Brimblecombe, N., Moriarty, J., Damant, J., Knapp, M. and Manthorpe, J. (2021) Supporting carers following the implementation of the Care Act 2014: Eligibility, support and prevention: The Carers in Adult Social Care (CASC) study. Report, LSE and NIHR Policy Research Unit in Health and Social Care Workforce.

Finch, J. and Groves, D. (1983) *A Labour of Love: Women, Work, and Caring*. Abingdon: Routledge.

Fine, M.. (2007) *A Caring Society? Care and the Dilemmas of Human Services in the 21st Century*. Basingstoke: Macmillan International Higher Education.

Fine, M. (2020) Reconstructing dependency: Precarity, precariousness and care in old age. In A. Grenier, C. Phillipson and R.A. Settersten Jr (eds) *Precarity and Ageing: Understanding Insecurity and Risk in Later Life*. Bristol: Policy Press, pp 169–190.

Fisher, B. and Tronto, J. (1991) Towards a feminist theory of care. In E. Abel and M. Nelson (eds) *Circles of Care: Work and Identity in Women's Lives*. New York: University of New York Press.

Fraser, N. (2009) *Scales of Justice: Reimagining Political Space in a Globalizing World*. New York: Columbia University Press.

George, M. (2001) *It Could Be You: A Report on the Chances of Becoming a Carer*. London: Carers UK.

Gillard, J. (2014) *My Story*. Camberwell: Random House Australia.

Gillies, B. (2000) Acting up: Role ambiguity and the legal recognition of carers. *Ageing & Society*, 20(4), 429–444.

Gilligan, C. (1993) *In a Different Voice*. Cambridge, MA: Harvard University Press.

Glendinning, C. (1986) *A Single Door: Social Work with the Families of Disabled Children*. London: Allen & Unwin.

Glendinning, C., Challis, D.J., Fernández, J.-L., Jacobs, S., Jones, K., Knapp, M., Manthorpe, J., Moran, N., Netten, A. and Stevens, M. (2008) *Evaluation of the Individual Budgets Pilot Programme*. Final Report. York: Social Policy Research Unit, University of York.

Glendinning, C., Mitchell, W. and Brooks, J. (2015) Ambiguity in practice? Carers' roles in personalised social care in England. *Health & Social Care in the Community*, 23(1), 23–32.

Glennon, R., Hodgkinson, I., Knowles, J., Radnor, Z. and Bateman, N. (2018) Public sector 'modernisation': Examining the impact of a change agenda on local government employees in England. *Australian Journal of Public Administration*, 77(2), 203–221.

Godfrey, M. and Townsend, J. (2009) Delayed hospital discharge in England and Scotland: A comparative study of policy and implementation. *Journal of Integrated Care*, 17(1), 26–36.

Government Office for Science (2016) Future of an ageing population. In *The Foresight Report*. London: Government Office for Science.

Graham, H. (1983) Caring: A labour of love. In J. Finch and D. Groves (eds) *A Labour of Love: Women, Work and Caring*. London: Routledge and Keegan Paul, pp 3–30.

Green, H. (1988) *General Household Survey 1985: Informal Carers*. London: HMSO.

Greenwood, N., Habibi, R. and Mackenzie, A. (2012) Respite: Carers' experiences and perceptions of respite at home. *BMC Geriatrics*, 12(42), 1–12.

Grenier, A., Lloyd, L. and Phillipson, C. (2017) Precarity in late life: Rethinking dementia as a 'frailed' old age. *Sociology of Health & Illness*, 39(2), 318–330.

Grenier, A., Phillipson, C. and Stetterson, R.A. Jr (2020) Precarity and ageing: New perspectives for social gerontology. In A. Grenier, C. Phillipson and R.A. Stettersen Jr (eds) *Precarity and Ageing: Understanding Insecurity and Risk in Later Life*. Bristol: Policy Press, pp 1–2.

Griffiths, R. (1988) *Community Care, the Agenda for Action* [also known as The Griffiths Report]. London: HMSO.

Ham, C., Heenan, D., Longley, M. and Steel, D.R. (2013) *Integrated Care in Northern Ireland, Scotland and Wales: Lessons for England*. London: The King's Fund.

Hamilton, S., Szymczynska, P., Clewett, N., Manthorpe, J., Tew, J., Larsen, J. and Pinfold, V. (2017) The role of family carers in the use of personal budgets by people with mental health problems. *Health & Social Care in the Community*, 25(1), 158–166.

Hankivsky, O. (2005) *Social Policy and the Ethic of Care*. Vancouver: University of British Columbia Press.

Hankivsky, O. (2014) Rethinking care ethics: On the promise and potential of intersectional analysis. *American Political Science Review*, 108(2), 252–264.

Hansard (1995a) [HC] Volume 258, April 1995 Assessment and Provision of Carers' Services.

Hansard (1995b) [HL] Volume 564, cc628–634, House of Lords Debate, 17 May 1995.

Hansard (1996) [HC] Volume 571, cc752–782, Disabled Persons and Carers (Short Term Breaks).

Hansard (1998) [HL] Volume 308, cc1305–1307, Disabled Persons and Carers: Short Term Breaks Bill.

Hansard (2000) [HC] Volume 343, cc1336–1398, Carers and Disabled Children Bill.

Hansard (2004) Vol 421, c573 Carers (Equal Opportunities) Bill.

Hansard (2018) [HC] Early Day Motion 1814.

Hansard (2021) [HC] 12-3-2021 at 14.38 Barbara Keeley.

Haw-Wells, J. (2017) Informal carers' opinions on the Care Programme Approach in mental health. *Nursing Times*, 113(10), 53–56.

Heenan, D. (2000) Informal care in farming families in Northern Ireland: Some considerations for social work. *British Journal of Social Work*, 30, 855–866.

Henwood, M., Larkin, M. and Milne, A. (2019) *Seeing the Wood for the Trees. Carer Related Research and Knowledge: A Scoping Review*. London: NIHR School for Social Care Research.

Hepworth, D. (2005) Asian carers' perceptions of care assessment and support in the community. *British Journal of Social Work*, 35(3), 337–353.

Heron, C. (1998) *Working with Carers*. London: Jessica Kingsley.

Herring, J. (2014) The disability critique of care. *Elder Law Review*, 8, 1–15.

Hervey, N. and Ramsay, R. (2004) Carers as partners in care. *Advances in Psychiatric Treatment*, 10(2), 81–84.

Hirst, M. (2001) Trends in informal care in Great Britain during the 1990s. *Health & Social Care in the Community*, 9(6), 348–357.

HM Government (1999a) *Caring about Carers: A National Strategy for Carers*. London: HM Government.

HM Government (1999b) *A Real Break: Guidebook on the Provision of Short Term Breaks*. London: HM Government.

HM Government (2008) *Carers at the Heart of 21st Century Families and Communities: 'A Caring System on Your Side. A Life of Your Own'*. London: HM Government.

HM Government (2010) *Recognised, Valued and Supported: Next Steps for the Carers Strategy*. London: HM Government.

Hochschild, A.R. (2003) *The Commercialization of Intimate Life: Notes from Home and Work*. Oakland: University of California Press.

Holzhausen, E. and Jackson A. (1997a) *Still Battling? The Carers Act One Year On*. London: Carers National Association.

Holzhausen, E. and Jackson, A. (1997b) *In on the Act? Social Services' Experience of the First Year of the Carers Act*. London: Carers National Association.

House of Commons (1990) *Session 1989–90 Social Services Committee Report. Community Care: Carers*.

House of Commons (1994) Carers (Recognition and Services) Bill.

House of Commons (1996) Disabled Persons and Carers (Short Term Breaks) Bill.

House of Commons (2007) Carers (Identification and Support) Bill.

House of Commons (2009) Session 2008–2009 Report by the Comptroller and Auditor General Supporting Carers to Care.

House of Commons (2018a) Thirteenth Report of Session 2017–2019 Work and Pensions Select Committee HC581 Employment Support for Carers.

House of Commons (2018b) Employment Support for Carers: Government Response to the Committee's Thirteenth Report HC1463.

House of Commons Work and Pensions Committee (2008a) Fourth Report of Session 2007–8. Volume 2 Oral and Written Evidence.

House of Commons Work and Pensions Committee (2018b) Employment Support for Carers: Government Response to the Committee's Thirteenth Report. Thirteenth Special Report of Session 2017–2019 HC1463.

Hudson, B. (2021) *Clients, Consumers or Citizens? The Privatisation of Adult Social Care in England*. Bristol: Policy Press.

Hudson, B. and Henwood, M. (2002) The NHS and social care: The final countdown? *Policy & Politics*, 30(2), 153–166.

Hudson-Sharp, N., Munro-Lott, N., Rolfe, H. and Runge, J. (2018) The impact of welfare reform and welfare-to-work programmes: An evidence review. *Research Report 111*. Equality and Human Rights Commission.

Humphrey, J.C. (2003) New Labour and the regulatory reform of social care. *Critical Social Policy*, 23(1), 5–24.

Isham, L., Bradbury-Jones, C. and Hewison, A. (2020) Female family carers' experiences of violent, abusive or harmful behaviour by the older person for whom they care: A case of epistemic injustice? *Sociology of Health & Illness*, 42(1), 80–94.

James, G. (2016) Family-friendly employment laws (re) assessed: The potential of care ethics. *Industrial Law Journal*, 45(4), 477–502.

Jepson, A. (2020) Adult social care and support in Scotland. *SPICe Briefing/Pàipear-ullachaidh SPICe*. The Scottish Parliament.

Jepson, M., Laybourne, A., Williams, V., Cyhlarova, E., Williamson, T. and Jessiman, T. and Lloyd, L. (2018) Hard times for older carers and older people. Paper presented at the Annual Conference of the British Society of Gerontology, 4–6 July, Manchester.

Jones, R. (2021) *A History of the Personal Social Services in England: Feast, Famine and the Future*. Cham: Palgrave Macmillan.

Katbamna, S., Ahmad, W., Bhakta, P., Baker, R. and Parker, G. (2004) Do they look after their own? Informal support for South Asian carers. *Health & Social Care in the Community*, 12(5), 398–406.

Katz, S. (2020) Precarious life, human development and the life course: Critical intersections. In A. Grenier, C. Phillipson and R.A. Settersten Jr (eds) *Precarity and Ageing*. Bristol: Policy Press, pp 41–66.

Kelly, D. and Kennedy, J. (2017) *Power to People: Proposals to Reboot Adult Social Care and Support in Northern Ireland*. Expert Advisory Panel on Adult Care and Support. Belfast: Department of Health/An Roinn Sláinte/Männystrie o Poustie.

Kendall, J., Mohan, J., Brookes, N. and Yoon, Y. (2018) The English voluntary sector: How volunteering and policy climate perceptions matter. *Journal of Social Policy*, 47(4), 759–782.

Ketola, M. and Hughes, C. (2018) Changing narratives, changing relationships: A new environment for voluntary action? *Voluntary Sector Review*, 9(2), 197–214.

King's Fund (1997) *Carers Impact: How Do We Know When We Have Got There? Improving Support to Carers: Report of the First Year's Work of Carers Impact*. London: King's Fund.

King's Fund (1999) *The Carers Compass: Directions for Improving Support for Carers*. London: King's Fund.

Kittay, E.F. (1999) *Love's Labor: Essays on Women, Equality, and Dependency*. New York: Routledge.

Kittay, E.F. (2011) The ethics of care, dependence and disability. *Ratio Juris*, 24(1), 49–58.

Kohner, N. (1993) *A Stronger Voice: The Achievements of the Carer's Movement 1963–1993*. London: Carers National Association.

Kröger, T. (2022) *Care Poverty: When Older People's Needs Remain Unmet*. Cham: Springer Nature.

Land, H. (1978) Who cares for the family? *Journal of Social Policy*, 7(3), 257–284.

Lanoix, M. (2013) Labor as embodied practice: The lessons of care work. *Hypatia*, 28(1), 85–100.

Larkin, M. and Mitchell, W. (2016) Carers, choice and personalisation: What do we know? *Social Policy and Society*, 15(2), 189–205.

Larkin, M., Henwood, M. and Milne, A. (2019) Carer-related research and knowledge: Findings from a scoping review. *Health & Social Care in the Community*, 27(1), 55–67.

Leece, J. (2002) Extending direct payments to informal carers: Some issues for local authorities. *Practice*, 14(2), 31–44.

Lewis, T. (2016) *Flexible Working: Legal Rights and Gaps in the Law*. London, UNISON.

LGA (Local Government Association) (2021) LGA Response to White Paper: 'People at the heart of care: adult social care reform', 30 December. London: LGA.

Lipsky, M. (1980) *Street Level Bureaucracy*. New York: Russell Sage Foundation.

Lipsky, M. (2010) *Street-Level Bureaucracy: Dilemmas of the Individual in Public Service*. New York: Russell Sage Foundation.

Llewellyn, M., Verity, F., Wallace, S. and Tetlow, S. (2022) Expectations and experiences: Service user and carer perspectives on the Social Services and Well-being (Wales) Act. *Social Research number 16/2022*. Welsh Government/Llywodraeth Cymru.

References

Lloyd, L. (2000) Caring about carers: Only half the picture? *Critical Social Policy*, 20(1), 136–150.

Lloyd, L. (2004) Mortality and morality: Ageing and the ethics of care. *Ageing & Society*, 24(2), 235–256.

Lloyd, L. (2006) Call us carers: Limitations and risks in campaigning for recognition and exclusivity. *Critical Social Policy*, 26(4), 945–960.

Lloyd, L. (2020) Devalued later life: Older residents' experiences of risk in a market system of residential and nursing homes. In P. Armstrong and H. Armstrong (eds) *The Privatization of Care: The Case of Nursing Homes*. Abingdon: Routledge, pp 196–208.

Lloyd, L. and Jessiman, T. (2017) 'They gave us this leaflet...': Older people's experience of providing personal care for partners. Paper presented at the British Society of Gerontology 46th Annual Conference, 5–7 July, Swansea.

Lloyd, L., Tanner, D., Milne, A., Ray, M., Richards S., Sullivan M.P., Beech, C. and Phillips, J. (2014) Look after yourself: Active ageing, individual responsibility and the decline of social work with older people. *European Journal of Social Work*, 17(3), 322–335.

Lloyd, L., Jessiman, T., Cameron, A. and Bezzina, A. (2020) Support for older carers of older people: The 2014 Care Act. Webinar presentation, NIHR School for Social Care Research.

Lowndes, V. and Gardner, A. (2016) Local governance under the conservatives: Super-austerity, devolution and the 'smarter state'. *Local Government Studies*, 42(3), 357–375.

Lynch, K. (2021) *Care and Capitalism*. Cambridge: Polity Press.

MacKinnon, D. (2015) Devolution, state restructuring and policy divergence in the UK. *The Geographical Journal*, 181(1), 47–56.

Mackley, A. and McInnes, R. (2020) Social security powers in the UK. Briefing Paper 9048, 9 November. House of Commons Library.

Maher, J. and Green, H. (2002) *Carers 2000: Results from the Carers Module of the General Household Survey 2000*. London: Stationery Office.

Mandelstam, M. (1999) *Community Care Practice and the Law*. London: Jessica Kingsley.

Manthorpe, J., Fernandez, J.L., Brimblecombe, N., Knapp, M., Snell, T. and Moriarty, J. (2019) Great expectations: Ambitions for family carers in UK parliamentary debates on the Care Bill. *International Journal of Care and Caring*, 3(3), 359–374.

Marczak, J., Fernandez, J.L., Manthorpe, J., Brimblecombe, N., Moriarty, J., Knapp, M. and Snell, T. (2021) How have the Care Act 2014 ambitions to support carers translated into local practice? Findings from a process evaluation study of local stakeholders' perceptions of Care Act implementation. *Health & Social Care in the Community*, 30(5), 1711–1720.

May, P.J. (2015) Implementation failures revisited: Policy regime perspectives. *Public Policy and Administration*, 30(3–4), 277–299.

Means, R. and Smith, R. (1998) *From Poor Law to Community Care: The Development of Welfare Services for Elderly People 1939–1971*. 2nd edition. Bristol: Policy Press.

Means, R., Morbey, H. and Smith, R. (2002) *From Community Care to Market Care? The Development of Welfare Services for Older People*. Bristol: Policy Press.

Means, R., Richards, S. and Smith, R. (2003) *Community Care: Policy and Practice*. 3rd edition. Basingstoke: Macmillan International Higher Education.

Milne, A. (2020) *Mental Health in Later Life: Taking a Life Course Approach*. Bristol: Policy Press.

Milne, A. and Larkin, M. (2015) Knowledge generation about care-giving in the UK: A critical review of research paradigms. *Health & Social Care in the Community*, 23(1), 4–13.

Mitchell, W., Brooks, J. and Glendinning, C. (2014) Personalisation: Where do carers fit? In C. Needham and J. Glasby (eds) *Debates in Personalisation*. Bristol: Policy Press, pp 65–74.

Mooney, G., Scott, G. and Williams, C. (2006) *Introduction: Rethinking Social Policy through Devolution*. London, Thousand Oaks and New Delhi: SAGE.

Moran, N., Arksey, H., Glendinning, C., Jones, K., Netten, A. and Rabiee, P. (2012) Personalisation and carers: Whose rights? Whose benefits? *British Journal of Social Work*, 42(3), 461–479.

Morgan, F. (2018) The treatment of informal care-related risks as social risks: An analysis of the English care policy system. *Journal of Social Policy*, 47(1), 179–196.

Morgan, R. (2002) Clear red water. Speech by the First Minister for Wales to the National Centre for Public Policy, Swansea.

Morgan, T., Duschinsky, R., Gott, M. and Barclay, S. (2021) Problematising carer identification: A narrative study with older partner's providing end-of-life care. *SSM-Qualitative Research in Health*, 1, 100015.

Moriarty, J. and Manthorpe, J. (2014) Fragmentation and competition: Voluntary organisations' experiences of support for family carers. *Voluntary Sector Review*, 5(2), 249–257.

Moriarty, J., Manthorpe, J. and Cornes, M. (2015) Reaching out or missing out: Approaches to outreach with family carers in social care organisations. *Health & Social Care in the Community*, 23(1), 42–50.

Morris, J. (1993) *Independent Lives? Community Care and Disabled People*. London: Red Globe Press.

National Assembly for Wales (2000) *Caring about Carers: The Carers Strategy in Wales – Implementation Plan*. Cardiff: National Assembly for Wales.

National Assembly for Wales (2010) Carers Strategies (Wales) Measure 2010 nawm5 (original version). Cardiff: National Assembly for Wales.

National Assembly for Wales (2014) Social Services and Well-Being (Wales) Act, 2104 anaw4. Cardiff: National Assembly for Wales.

National Assembly for Wales – Health Social Care and Sport Committee (2019) *Caring for our Future: An Inquiry into the Impact of the Social Services and Wellbeing (Wales) Act 2014 in Relation to Carers*. Cardiff: National Assembly for Wales Commission.

National Audit Office (2015) Care Act first-phase reforms. *Report by the Comptroller and Auditor General*. Department of Health HC82n Session 2015–2016, 11 June.

National Health Service (NHS) Education for Scotland (2013) Equal Partners in Care (EPIC): Practice Guidance for working with carers and young carers. NHS Education for Scotland and Scottish Social Services Council. Edinburgh: NHS Education for Scotland.

National Institute for Health and Care Excellence (NICE) (2021) *Supporting Adult Carers: Quality Standard*. National Institute for Health and Care Excellence. Available at: www.nice.orh.uk/guidance/qs200

NCO (National Carer Organisations) (2020) NCO response to Scottish Parliament Health and Sport Committee call for written evidence to the Social Care Inquiry. National Carer Organisations.

Needham, C. (2012) *What is Happening to Day Centre Services? Voices From Frontline Staff*. UNISON and University of Birmingham Health Services Management Centre. London: UNISON.

Needham, C. and Dickinson, H. (2018) 'Any one of us could be among that number': Comparing the policy narratives for individualized disability funding in Australia and England. *Social Policy & Administration*, 52(3), 731–749.

Needham, C. and Glasby, J. (2014) Taking stock of personalisation. In C. Needham and J. Glasby (eds) *Debates in Personalisation*. Bristol: Policy Press, pp 11–24.

NIHRC (Northern Ireland Human Rights Commission) (2014) *The Human Rights of Carers in Northern Ireland*. Belfast: Northern Ireland Human Rights Commission.

Noddings, N. (1984) *Caring: A feminine approach to ethics*. Oakland: University of California Press.

Nolan, M., Grant, G. and Keady, J. (1996) *Understanding Family Care: A Multidimensional Model of Caring and Coping*. Buckingham: Open University Press.

Northern Ireland Assembly (2001) Speech by Mark Durkan, Minister of Finance and Personnel. Debate on Alternatives to Private Finance Initiatives/Public-Private Partnerships, 1 October.

O'Rourke, G., Lloyd, L., Bezzina, A., Cameron, A., Jessiman, T. and Smith, R. (2021) Supporting older co-resident carers of older people: The impact of Care Act implementation in four local authorities in England. *Social Policy and Society*, 20(3), 371–384.

ONS (2013) 2011 Census analysis: Unpaid care in England and Wales, 2011 and comparison with 2001. London: Office for National Statistics.

Older People's Commissioner for Wales (2018) Response from the Older People's Commissioner for Wales to National Assembly for Wales, Health, Social Care and Sport Committee: Inquiry into the impact of the Social Services and Wellbeing (Wales) Act 2014 in relation to carers. Cardiff: Office of the Older People's Commissioner for Wales.

Olsen, R., Parker, G. and Drewett, A. (1997) Carers and the missing link: Changing professional attitudes. *Health & Social Care in the Community*, 5(2), 116–123.

Parker, G. (1990) With due care and attention: A review of research on informal care. *Occasional Paper 2*. London: Family Policy Studies Centre.

Parker, G. (1993) *With this Body: Caring and Disability in Marriage*. Buckingham: Open University Press.

Parker, G. (1994) *Where Next for Research on Carers?* Leicester: University of Leicester, Nuffield Community Care Studies Unit.

Parker, G. (1999) Impact of the NHS and Community Care Act (1990) on informal carers. Royal Commission on Long Term Care with Respect to Old Age. Cm 4192-II.123, March.

Parker, G. and Clarke, H. (2002) Making the ends meet: Do carers and disabled people have a common agenda? *Policy & Politics*, 30(3), 347–359.

Parker, G. and Lawton, D. (1994) *Different Types of Care, Different Types of Carer: Evidence from the General Household Survey*. London: HMSO.

Parker, G., Arksey, H. and Harden, M. (2010) *Meta-Review of International Evidence on Interventions to Support Carers*. York: Social Policy Research Unit, University of York.

Parsloe, P. (1993) Making a bid for fair play. *Community Care*, 5 August, pp 16–17.

Petrie, K. and Kirkup, J. (2018) *Caring for Carers*. London: The Social Market Foundation.

Pickard, L. (2001) Carer break or carer-blind? Policies for informal carers in the UK. *Social Policy & Administration*, 35(4), 441–458.

Pickard, L. (2012) Substitution between formal and informal care: A 'natural experiment' in social policy in Britain between 1985 and 2000. *Ageing and Society*, 32(7), 1147–1175.

Pickard, L., Wittenberg, R., Comas-Herrera, A., Davies, B. and Darton, R. (2000) Relying on informal care in the new century? Informal care for elderly people in England to 2031. *Ageing & Society*, 20(6), 745–772.

Pickard, L., Brimblecombe, N., King, D. and Knapp, M. (2018) 'Replacement care' for working carers? A longitudinal study in England, 2013–15. *Social Policy & Administration*, 52(3), 690–709.

Pickard, S. (2010) The 'good carer': Moral practices in late modernity. *Sociology*, 44(3), 471–487.

References

Pitkeathley, J. (1989) *It's My Duty, Isn't It? The Plight of Carers in Our Society*. London: Souvenir Press.

Polanyi, K. (2001 [1944]) *The Great Transformation*. Boston: Beacon.

Pollock, K., Wilkinson, S., Perry-Young, L., Turner, N. and Schneider, J. (2021) What do family care-givers want from domiciliary care for relatives living with dementia? A qualitative study. *Ageing & Society*, 41(9), 2060–2073.

Pressman, J.L. and Wildavsky, A. (1984) *Implementation: How Great Expectations in Washington are Dashed in Oakland*. Berkeley: University of California Press.

PRTC and ADASS (Princess Royal Trust for Carers and Association of Directors of Adult Social Services) (2010) *Supporting Carers: Early Interventions and Better Outcomes*. London: Princess Royal Trust for Carers and Association of Directors of Adult Social Services.

Pyper, D. (2018) Flexible working. Briefing Paper 01086, 3 October. London, House of Commons Library.

Rand, S. and Malley, J. (2014) Carers' quality of life and experiences of adult social care support in England. *Health & Social Care in the Community*, 22(4), 375–385.

Rand, S., Malley J. and Forder, J. (2019) Are reasons for care-giving related to carers' care-related quality of life and strain? Evidence from a survey of carers in England. *Health and Social Care in the Community*, 27, 151–160.

Rawls, J. (1971) *A Theory of Justice*. Cambridge, MA: Harvard University Press.

Rhodes, R.A. (1997) *Understanding Governance: Policy Networks, Governance, Reflexivity and Accountability*. Buckingham: Open University.

Rhodes, R.A. (2007) Understanding governance: Ten years on. *Organization Studies*, 28(8), 1243–1264.

Robinson, C. and Williams, V. (2002) Carers of people with learning disabilities, and their experience of the 1995 Carers Act. *British Journal of Social Work*, 32(2), 169–183.

Rosenfeld, D., Bartlam, B. and Smith R.D. (2012) Out of the closet and into the trenches: Gay male baby boomers, aging and HIV/AIDS. *The Gerontologist*, 52(2), 255–264.

Royal Commission on Long Term Care (1999) *With Respect to Old Age: Long Term Care: Rights and Responsibilities*. Cm 4192-I, March. London: The Stationery Office.

Rummery, K. and Fine, M. (2012) Care: A critical review of theory, policy and practice. *Social Policy & Administration*, 46(3), 321–343.

Sandel, M.J. (2012) *What Money Can't Buy: The Moral Limits of Markets*. Basingstoke: Macmillan.

Sayer, A. (2005) Class, moral worth and recognition. *Sociology*, 39(5), 947–963.

Sayer, A. (2011) *Why Things Matter to People: Social Science, Values and Ethical Life*. Cambridge: Cambridge University Press.

SCIE (Social Care Institute for Excellence) (2007) *Social Care Institute for Excellence Guide 9: Implementing the Carers (Equal Opportunities) Act 2004*. London: SCIE.

Scottish Care Inspectorate (2020) Carers (Scotland) Act 2016 Policy and Legislation Carers.

Scottish Government (1999) *Strategy for Carers in Scotland*. Edinburgh: Scottish Government.

Scottish Government (2010) *Caring Together: The Carers Strategy for Scotland 2010–2015*. Edinburgh: Scottish Government.

Scottish Government/Riaghaltas na h-Alba (2018) *Carers' Charter: Your Rights as an Adult Carer or Young Carer in Scotland*. Edinburgh: Scottish Government.

Scottish Government/Riaghaltas na h-Alba (2021) *Carers (Scotland) Act 2016: Statutory Guidance*. Edinburgh: Scottish Government.

Scottish Parliament (1999) Official Report 25 Nov column 1012. 15.50. Meeting of the Parliament.

Scourfield, P. (2005) Understanding why carers' assessments do not always take place. *Practice*, 17(1), 15–28.

Seddon, D. and Prendergast, L. (2019) *Short Breaks for Carers: A Scoping Review*. Bangor: Wales Centre for Ageing and Dementia Research, Bangor University / Shared Care Scotland.

Seddon, D. and Robinson, C.A. (2001) Carers of older people with dementia: assessment and the Carers Act. *Health and Social Care in the Community*, 9(3), 151–158.

Seddon, D. and Robinson, C. (2015) Carer assessment: Continuing tensions and dilemmas for social care practice. *Health & Social Care in the Community*, 23(1), 14–22.

Seddon, D., Robinson, C., Reeves, C., Tommis, Y., Woods, B. and Russell, I. (2007) In their own right: Translating the policy of carer assessment into practice. *British Journal of Social Work*, 37(8), 1335–1352.

Seddon, D., Robinson, C., Tommis, Y., Woods, B., Perry, J. and Russell, I. (2010) A study of the carers strategy (2000): Supporting carers in Wales. *British Journal of Social Work*, 40(5), 1470–1487.

Sevenhuijsen, S. (1998) *Citizenship and the Ethics of Care: Feminist Considerations on Justice, Morality and Politics*. London: Routledge.

Sevenhuijsen, S. (2000) Caring in the third way: The relation between obligation, responsibility and care in Third Way discourse. *Critical Social Policy*, 20(1), 5–37.

Shakespeare, T. (2006) *Disability Rights and Wrongs*. 1st edition. London: Routledge.

Shakespeare, T. (2013) *Disability Rights and Wrongs Revisited*. London: Routledge.

Shaw, E., Nunns, M., Briscoe, S., Anderson, R. and Thompson Coon, J. (2018) Experiences of the 'Nearest Relative' provisions in the compulsory detention of people under the Mental Health Act: Rapid systematic review. *Health Services and Delivery Research*, 6(39).

Simpson, A., Miller, C. and Bowers, L.E.N. (2003) The history of the Care Programme Approach in England: Where did it go wrong? *Journal of Mental Health*, 12(5), 489–504.

Smith, M.S. (2015) 'Only connect': 'Nearest relative's' experiences of mental health act assessments. *Journal of Social Work Practice*, 29(3), 339–353.

Smith, R., Lloyd, L., Cameron, A., Johnson, E. and Willis, P. (2019) What is (adult) social care in England? Its origins and meaning. *Research, Policy and Planning*, 33(2), 45–56.

Social Services Inspectorate (SSI) (1995) *Caring Today: A National Inspection of Local Authority Support to Carers*. London: DH.

Social Services Inspectorate (SSI) (1998) *A Matter of Chance for Carers? Inspection of Local Authority Support for Carers*. London: DH.

Social Services Inspectorate/Social Work (Services Group) (SSI/SWSG) (1991) *Care Management and Assessment: Practitioners' Guide*. London: HMSO.

Stalker, K. and Campbell, I. (2002) *Review of Care Management in Scotland (Health and Community Care Research Findings)*. Edinburgh: Scottish Executive.

Standing, G. (2011) The precariat: From denizens to citizens? *Polity*, 44(4), 558–608.

Stensöta, H.O. (2020) Democratic care 'for all' and trade-offs: The public solution, civil society and the market. *International Journal of Care and Caring*, 4(1), 75–89.

Stratton, A. and Pearse, D. (2010) Audit watchdog axed by Pickles in austerity drive. *The Guardian*, 13 August.

Taylor, B.J. (2012) Developing an integrated assessment tool for the health and social care of older people. *British Journal of Social Work*, 42, 1293–1314.

Templeton, F., Mitchell, D. and Luff, R. (2021) *Review of Evidence Relating to Unpaid Carer's Needs Assessments in Wales*. London: Social Care Institute for Excellence.

Thomas, C. (1993) De-constructing concepts of care. *Sociology*, 27(4), 649–669.

Thomas, C. (2007) *Sociologies of Disability and Illness: Contested Ideas in Disability Studies and Medical Sociology*. Basingstoke: Palgrave Macmillan.

Thomas, S., Dalton, J., Harden, M., Eastwood, A. and Parker, G. (2017) Updated meta-review of evidence on support for carers. *Health Services and Delivery Research*, 5(12).

Tonks, A. (1994) Community care: The first year. Community care in Northern Ireland: A promising start. *BMJ*, 308(6932), 839–842.

Tronto, J. (1993) *Moral Boundaries: A Political Argument for an Ethic of Care*. New York: Routledge.

Tronto, J. (2010) Creating caring institutions: Politics, plurality and purpose. *Ethics and Social Welfare*, 4(2), 158–171.

Tronto, J. (2013) *Caring Democracy: Markets, Equality and Justice*. New York: New York University Press.

Tronto, J. (2017) There is an alternative: Homines curans and the limits of neoliberalism. *International Journal of Care and Caring*, 1(1), 27–43.

Turnpenny, A., Rand, S., Whelton, B., Beadle-Brown, J. and Babaian, J. (2021) Family carers managing personal budgets for adults with learning disabilities or autism. *British Journal of Learning Disabilities*, 49(1), 52–61.

Twigg, J. (2000) Carework as a form of bodywork. *Ageing & Society*, 20(4), 389–411.

Twigg, J. and Atkin, K. (1994) *Carers Perceived: Policy and Practice in Informal Care*. Buckingham: Open University.

UN (United Nations) (1995) *Report of the Fourth World Conference on Women. Beijing, 4–15 September 1995*. Geneva: United Nations.

UN (United Nations) (2017) Convention on the Rights of Persons with Disabilities. Committee on the Rights of Persons with Disabilities. *Concluding observations on the initial report of the United Kingdom of Great Britain and Northern Ireland*. CRPD/C/GBR/CO1. Geneva: United Nations.

Waerness, K. (2018) Social research, political theory and the ethics of care in a global perspective. In T.R. Eriksen (ed) *Dilemmas of Care in the Nordic Welfare State: Continuity and Change*. London Routledge, pp 15–30.

Walker, A. (1982) *Public Expenditure and Social Policy*. London: Heinemann.

Walker, A. (1994) *Half a Century of Promises: The Failure to Realise 'Community Care' for Older People*. London: Counsel and Care.

Walker, A. (1995) Integrating the family into a mixed economy of care. In I. Allen and E. Perkins (eds) *The Future of Family Care for Older People*. London: HMSO, pp 201–220.

Warner, N. (1995) *Better Tomorrows: Report of a National Study of Carers and the Community Care Changes*. London: Carers National Association.

Watson, N., McKie, L., Hughes, B., Hopkins, D. and Gregory, S. (2004) (Inter) dependence, needs and care: The potential for disability and feminist theorists to develop an emancipatory model. *Sociology*, 38(2), 331–350.

Welsh Assembly Government (2000) *Caring About Carers: The Carers Strategy in Wales, Implementation Plan*. Cardiff: Welsh Assembly Government. Cardiff

Welsh Government/Llywodraeth Cymru (2003) *Challenging the Myth 'They Look after Their Own'*. Cardiff: Welsh Government.

Welsh Government/Llywodraeth Cymru (2011) *Carers Strategies (Wales) Measure 2010: Guidance Issued to Local Health Boards and Local Authorities*. Cardiff: Welsh Government.

Welsh Government/Llywodraeth Cymru (2021) *Strategy for Unpaid Carers*. WG42215. Cardiff: Welsh Government.

Wiles, J. (2011) Reflections on being a recipient of care: Vexing the concept of vulnerability. *Social and Cultural Geography*, 12, 573–588.

Williams, C. and Mooney, G. (2008) Decentring social policy? Devolution and the discipline of social policy: A commentary. *Journal of Social Policy*, 37(3), 489–507.

Williams, F. (2001) in and beyond New Labour: Towards a new political ethics of care. *Critical Social Policy*, 21(4), 467–493.

Williams, F. (2010) Claiming and framing in the making of care policies. *The Recognition and Redistribution of Care. Gender and Development Programme Paper 13*. United Nations Research Institute for Social Development.

Willis, P.B., Ward, N. and Fish, J. (2011) Searching for LGBT carers: Mapping a research agenda in social work and social care. *British Journal of Social Work*, 41(7), 1304–1320.

Willis, P.B., Lloyd, L.E., Bezzina, A. and Ali, B.B. (2021) Online advice to carers: An updated review of local authority websites in England. *Project Findings* NIHR School for Social Care Research. Available at: www.sscr.nihr.ac.uk/project-findings/

Wistow, G. (2005) Developing social care: The past, the present and the future. *Position Paper 04*. London: Social Care Institute for Excellence.

Woolham, J., Steils, N., Daly, G. and Ritters, K. (2018) The impact of personal budgets on unpaid carers of older people. *Journal of Social Work*, 18(2), 119–141.

Yeandle, S. (2016) Caring for our carers: An international perspective on policy developments in the UK. *Juncture*, 23(1), 57–62.

Yeandle, S. and Buckner, L. (2007) *Carers, Employment and Services: Time for a New Social Contract?* London: Carers UK and University of Leeds.

Young, H., Grundy, E. and Jitlal, M. (2006) *Care Providers, Care Receivers: A Longitudinal Perspective*. York: Joseph Rowntree Foundation.

Zhang, Y., Bennett, M. and Yeandle, S. (2019) *Will I Care? The Likelihood of Being a Carer in Adult Life*. London: Carers UK.

Index

A
abuse 84, 107
ageing population 4, 136
Alcock, P. 71
anti-care culture 125
Arber, S. 17, 19, 119
Arksey, H. 77–78, 82, 102, 103, 142
Ash, A. 84, 107
Association of Directors of Social Services (ADSS) 67, 68, 71
Audit Commission 44, 96
austerian realism 100
austerity 61–62, 136
austerity policies 41, 97–100
Ayres, S. 93
Azong, J.A. 110–111

B
background resources, carers as 73, 76, 81
Baldwin, S. 17–18
Bangladeshi community 23
Banks, P. 66
Barclay Report 76
Barnes, C. 90
Barnes, M. 105, 118, 130, 141
Beckett, C. 2, 118, 129
benefits for carers 59–60
  see also Carer's Allowance
Best Value Inspectorate 96
Betts, J. 56
Boateng, P. 42
Bowes, A. 69
breaks for carers see respite care
Brimblecombe, N. 98
British Household Panel Survey 21
Buckner, L. 59–60
Bytheway, B. 17, 20, 116

C
capitalism 125
care
  in the community 5–12, 17–18, 72
  conceptualisation of 116, 121–122, 124–125
  see also personal care; replacement care; respite care; social care; telecare; unpaid care
Care 21 49
Care Act, 2014 54–55
  carers' rights 110, 111
  perceptions of carers 138, 139
  practice guidance 70
  support for carers 85
  unpaid care as social risk 108–109
  welfare cuts 98
  whole family approach 140
care deficit 123–125, 132
care ethics see ethics of care
care management 7, 82
care poverty 125
Care Programme Approach 10, 69
'care receiving' 28
care relationships 2, 27, 34–35, 145
  conflict in 83–84
  feminist ethics of care 28–29, 31
  interdependence 118–119, 130
  routinisation of care services and 122
care services, routinisation of 121–123
caregiving 28
Carer Aware project 71
carer-blindness 25, 54, 75
carer-defined outcomes 46
carer identity 2–3, 76–79, 116, 137
carers
  definitions 13–14, 54, 55, 92
  emergence of term 17
  see also unpaid carers
carers' advisory groups 63
Carer's Allowance 43, 52, 53, 55, 59–60, 128
Carers and Direct Payments (Norther Ireland) Act, 2002 47
Carers and Disabled Children Act, 2000 45–46, 50, 68, 71, 81
'carers as experts' model 90
carers assessments 79–83, 94, 138–139, 140, 141
Carers at the Heart of 21st Century Families and Communities (HM Government 2008) 52, 128, 138
Carers Compass (King's Fund) 66
Carers (Equal Opportunities) Act, 2004 48, 49, 69, 78, 110
carers' groups / organisations
  Disabled Persons (Services, Consultation and Representation) Act, 1986 6
  grants for 85
  involvement in knowledge development 26
  involvement in policy development 16, 36, 64
  marginalisation of 141
  participation in local networks 105–106
  services offered by 72
  see also carers' advisory groups; Carers National Association; Carers Trust; Carers UK
carers' movement 5–6, 18, 20, 109

Index

Carers National Association 10, 26, 42, 67
  see also Carers UK
Carers (Recognition and Services) Act, 1995 36–40, 62, 67, 74, 81, 92, 102, 103
Carers Rights Charter 52, 111
Carers (Scotland) Act, 2016 56–57, 79, 139
Carers Strategies (Wales) Measures (National Assembly of Wales 2010) 53–54, 55, 63
Carers Strategy for Scotland 2010–2015 (Scottish Government 2010) 52–53
Carers Trust 26, 54, 72
Carers UK 42
  austerity 61, 98
  Children and Families Act, 2014 70
  cost-of-living crisis 60
  Employers for Carers 58
  numbers of unpaid carers 15, 24
  pressures experienced by unpaid carers 2
  unpaid care as economic opportunity 107–108
  unpaid caring as protected characteristic 49
  unpaid carers' priorities for social care reform 35, 129
  women as carers 18
Carers UK Northern Ireland 62
'caring about' 28, 124, 132
Caring about Carers: A National Strategy for Carers (HM Government 1999a) 42–43, 75, 78, 84–85
Caring about Carers: The Carers Strategy in Wales, Implementation Plan (Welsh Assembly Government 2000) 43–44
'caring for' 124, 132
Caring for People (DH 1989) 7, 8, 9, 11
'caring with' 29, 129
Carter, Lord 39
Census 2001 22–25, 42
children 98
Children and Families Act, 2014 58–59, 70
Clements, L. 48, 49, 51, 110, 111
Clough, B. 112, 130–131, 144–145
co-clients, carers as 73–74, 75, 86, 137, 138, 139
co-workers, carers as 73, 74, 75, 76, 86, 90, 137, 139
Coalition government 52, 58–59, 96, 98, 99, 105
Colebatch, H. 93, 101, 103
Coleman, S. 49
Coles, B. 89, 90
community care see care: in the community
Community Care: An Agenda for Action (Griffiths) 7
Community Care and Health (Scotland) Act, 2002 46–47
Community Care (Delayed Discharges) Act, 2003 46
Community Care (Direct Payments) Act, 1996 50
complex needs 79–80
conflict in care relationships 83–84
Conservative and Liberal Democrat Coalition government 52, 58–59, 96, 98, 99, 105
Conservative government 99, 100
contract culture 72
Cook, T. 6, 26, 76, 94
Cooper, C. 84
COVID-19 pandemic 15, 16, 62, 84, 93, 100, 106
Cramer, H. 89
Crossroad Care NI 72
Crossroads Care 72

D

Dahlberg, L. 23
Davey, E. 59
Davies, J.S. 100
Dayan, M. 56
delayed discharges 46
Delayed Discharges Action Plan 2002, Scotland 46
demographics 4, 136
dependency 31, 118–119, 120
  see also independence; interdependence
deprivation 23
devolution 40–41
  modernisation agenda and 96–97
  national strategies for carers 41–44
  see also individual nations
Dilnot, A. 1–2, 114
direct payments 27, 50, 53, 68, 86–87, 129
  anomaly in arrangements for 55
  independence and 118
  people with learning disabilities 51
  tension between unpaid and professional carers 89
disability rights movement 5–6, 27
disability rights perspective 74
disability, social model of 30
disabled people 14, 26, 90, 118
Disabled Persons and Carers (Short Term Breaks) Bill, 1996 39
Disabled Persons (Services, Consultation and Representation) Act, 1986 5–6
discrimination 49, 93
Drakeford, M. 99

E

Easton, D. 101
Eckersley, P. 99
economic and political contexts 95–100
economic opportunity, unpaid care as 107–108

Edwards, H. 39
Employers for Carers 58
employment 33
  austerity policies and 98
  as carer-defined outcome 46
  carers' rights agenda 48–49
  national strategies for carers 43, 44
  women 4, 22, 124
  see also flexible working
Employment Act, 2002 58
Employment (Reasonable Adjustments for Carers) Bill, 2020 59
employment rights 111–112
Employment Rights Act, 1996 58
England
  Carers Action Plan 2018–2020 61
  Carer's Allowance 59
  carers assessments 81
  carers' involvement 70
  numbers of unpaid carers 24
  policies to support carers **37–38**, 42–43, 45–46, 46, 52, 54–55
Equal Partners in Care (EPiC) 53
Equality Act, 2010 49–50, 59, 136–137
Equality Budgets 110–111
ethics of care 27–31, 116–117, 130–131, 132, 141
ethnic minority communities 23, 26, 47, 87
European Court of Justice 49
Exley, S. 105
experts, carers as 90

F

Family Resources Survey 15
Farnsworth, K. 98
feminist perspective 74
feminist research 17–18, 25, 26–27
  feminist ethics of care 27–31, 131
Fernandez, J.-L. 138, 139
Finch, J. 17
Fisher, B. 28
flexible working 58–59
Foresight Report 107
Francis, H. 48, 49
Fraser, N. 120, 123
'Future of an ageing population' (Government Office for Science) 107
Future of Unpaid Care in Scotland, The (Care 21) 49

G

gender *see* men as carers; women
General Household Surveys (GHS) 18–19, 21–22
Getting it Right for Carers (DH 1991) 9
Gillard, J. 127
Glendinning, C. 5
governance 104–106

Graham, H. 5
Greenwood, N. 89
Grenier, A. 119
Griffiths, R. 7, 74
Growing Older (DHSS 1981) 5
Growing the Care Market (Carers UK) 107–108

H

Hamilton, S. 89, 90
Hankivsky, O. 27, 30
Haw-Wells, J. 69
Heal, S. 103
Health Act, 1999 45
Heenan, D. 77
Henwood, M. 32–33, 34, 35
Hepworth, D. 77
Heron, C. 10, 74
Herring, J. 30–31
hidden carers 16, 32, 43, 76–77
Hirst, M. 21
Hochschild, A.R. 124–125, 126
home care services 9, 44, 88, 122, 129
Hudson, B. 95, 141
Hunt, J. 15

I

IBSEN study 50, 51
independence 27, 29, 31, 52, 118–119
  see also interdependence
individual budgets 50, 51, 127
inequalities, socioeconomic 98–99, 123
inter-relational risks 128
interdependence 27, 126, 127, 130
interest groups 99, 105
  see also carers' groups / organisations
Isham, L. 84

J

James, G. 111
Jepson, A. 24
joint working 102
  see also partnership working
justice 116–117, 144–145
  see also social justice

K

Katbamna, S. 77
Katz, S. 126, 140
Keeley, B. 61, 78
Ketola, M. 106
King's Fund 66, 71
Kittay, E.F. 31, 118
Kopel, A. and F. 46
Kröger, T. 125

L

Labour government
  carers as partners 95
  market economy in care 96

modernisation agenda 44–48, 96, 104–105
unpaid care as economic opportunity 107
unpaid care strategies and devolution 40–44
voluntary sector 106
Land, H. 5
Lanoix, M. 122
Larkin, M. 34
learning disabilities 46, 51, 67, 89
Leece, J. 86–87
legal system 130–131
Liberal Democrats 98, 103
Lipsky, M. 103–104
Llewellyn, M. 61–62, 100, 102
local authorities 99, 105
local service planning 70–73
Lowndes, V. 100
Lynch, K. 95, 123, 125

M

MacKinnon, D. 99
Maher, J. 21–22
Mandelstam, M. 10
Manthorpe, J. 106–107, 112
Marczak, J. 88
marital relationships 118
market economy 29, 96–97, 119, 139
May, P.J. 102
meaning making 103–104
see also unpaid care: framing in policies
Means, R. 4, 72
men as carers 18, 19, 21, 22, 23
mental health 10, 32–33, 44–45, 89
Milne, A. 34, 84
Mitchell, W. 81, 141
modernisation agenda 44–48, 96, 104–105
Morgan, F. 108–109, 127–128, 144
Morgan, T. 77
Moriarty, J. 72
Morris, J. 26
Mowat, D. 15

N

National Carer Organisation 61
National Disability Insurance Scheme (NDIS), Australia 127
National Service Frameworks (NSFs) 44–45
national strategies for carers 41–44
Needham, C. 127
needs assessments 79–83, 94, 138–139, 140, 141
neoliberal policies 121
neoliberalism 29, 95–96, 123, 125, 132
nested dependencies 31, 120
NHS and Community Care Act, 1990 3, 4–5, 7, 8, 9, 10, 20
Nolan, M. 25–26, 90
Northern Ireland 10
  Carer's Allowance 59

carers assessments 80
Crossroad Care NI 72
devolution 40–41, 97
numbers of unpaid carers 22
policies to support carers **37–38**, 44, 47–48, 54, 62
services and support for carers 68
Northern Ireland Human Rights Commission (NIHRC) 56, 137

O

Older Carers research project 72, 73, 80, 87, 99, 120, 122, 126
older people 119
Olsen, R. 16, 71
'Open Policy Making' 105
O'Rourke, G. 83, 109
outcomes 46, 66, 68, 82

P

Pakistani community 23
parent carers 68, 70, 89
Parker, G. 9, 11, 15, 19–20, 34, 85, 109, 111, 129, 136
Parsloe, P. 8
partnership working 105–106
  see also joint working
People First: Community Care in Northern Ireland in the 1990s (DHSS 1991) 10
personal budgets 50
personal care 20, 46, 85, 121–122, 129
personalisation agenda 50–51, 52, 63, 86
Petrie, K. 24
Pickard, L. 25, 75, 88, 97, 129
Pitkeathley, J. 3–4, 7, 20, 74, 85
Polanyi, K. 29
policy implementation 101–102
policy process 100–106
policy work 93
political and economic contexts 95–100
Pollock, K. 88, 139
population ageing 4, 136
positive outcomes focused approach 68, 82
postmodern stoicism 124, 125, 126
Practice Guidance 66–70, 74
precarity 119–120, 126–127, 131, 132, 143
prescription charges 41
Princess Royal Trust for Carers 71, 72
private carers 38
private sector care homes 6–7, 96
professionals, unpaid carers relationships with 89–91, 99
public spending *see* social care funding
Putting People First (DH 2007) 50–51

R

Rand, S. 88, 137
recognition 120–121, 132, 136–140
redistribution 120, 123

Redmond, I. 58
relationships *see* care relationships
replacement care 87, 88, 104, 142
resilience 126
respite care 39, 75, 87–89, 98, 103
Rix, Lord 39
Robinson, C. 67
Royal Commission on Long Term Care 75
Russell, P. 75

S

Sandel. M. 123
Sandwich Caring (Carers UK) 107
Sayer, A. 121, 140
Scotland 10
  austerity policies 99–100
  carers assessments 69, 80, 82
  carers' involvement 70
  carers' rights 49
  devolution 40, 41
  Equality Budgets 110–111
  modernisation agenda 96
  numbers of unpaid carers 24
  personal care 85
  policies to support carers **37–38**, 43, 46–47, 56–57
  social care inquiry 61
Scotland Act, 2016 59, 60
Scottish Carer's Assistance benefit 60
Scottish Census 24, 43
Scourfield, P. 81, 83, 84
Seddon, D. 46, 67, 69, 80, 82–83, 85, 88, 94
Seear, Baroness 39
Sevenhuijsen, S. 3, 30
Shakespeare, T. 30
Simpson, A. 69
sitting services 87
social care
  austerity policies and 97–100
  market economy in 96–97, 119
  routinisation of care services 121–123
social care costs 41
social care funding 1, 8, 41, 61, 97–100, 129
Social Care Institute for Excellence (SCIE) 69, 71, 78
social care policies 1
  see also unpaid care policies
social care reform 1–2, 54–57
  see also modernisation agenda
Social Care (Self-Directed Support) (Scotland) Act, 2013 53
social care systems 129–130, 132–133
social care workforce 99
  see also professionals, unpaid carers relationships with
social justice 99
Social Market Foundation 16, 24
social model of disability 30

social risk, unpaid care as 108–109, 127, 144
social services 123
Social Services and Wellbeing (Wales) Act, 2014 54, 55–56, 62, 100, 102, 139
Social Services Committee Report (House of Commons 1990) 6, 134
social workers 81, 84, 90, 141
Social Workers: Their Role and Tasks (Barclay, 1982) 76
socioeconomic conditions 120
socioeconomic inequalities 98–99, 123
Stalker, K. 82
State of Caring 2021 in Northern Ireland (Carers Northern Ireland 2021) 62
state, role of 36, 73, 92–93, 95–96, 127–129, 142–144
Stensöta, H.O. 129, 131, 143
stigma 123
Still Battling (Holzhausen and Jackson) 67
Strategy for Carers in Scotland (Scottish Government 1999) 43
Strategy for Learning Disabilities - Valuing People (DH 2001b) 46
street-level bureaucrats 103–104
superseded carers 74
Supporting Carers Today (DH 2018) 61

T

'taking care of' 28
technology 124
telecare 124, 125
Third Way 30, 40, 41
Thomas, C. 26–27, 129
Thomas, S. 85
Tonks, A. 10
Towards a Feminist Theory of Care (Fisher and Tronto) 28
Tronto, J. 28–30, 123, 129, 132, 141, 144
Turnpenny, A. 89
Twigg, J. 73, 83, 121, 141

U

unmet needs 138
unpaid care
  care relationships 2, 27, 34–35, 145
  conflict and 83–84
  feminist ethics of care 28–29, 31
  interdependence 118–119, 130
  routinisation of care services and 122
  Census 2001 question on 22–25
  current research 31–34
  debates and disputes in research 25–27
  as economic opportunity 107–108
  ethics of care 27–31, 116–117, 130–131
  formal care and 89–91, 99
  framing in policies 106–109, 123, 135–136
  knowledge development about 17–21
  marginalisation of 141–142
  patterns and trends in 21–22

perceived as widespread activity versus distinct category 115–121
as social risk 108–109, 127, 144
typology of 19–20
unpaid care policies **37–38**
 on carers' income 57–60
 carers' rights 48–51, 109–112, 136–137
 challenges 142–145
 devolution and 40–44
 economic and political contexts 95–100
 framing of unpaid care in 106–109, 123, 135–136
 historical perspective 3–5, 93–95
 impact of austerity and COVID-19 pandemic on 61–62
 implications of precarity for 125–131
 modernisation agenda and 44–48
 policy process 100–106
 potential and limitations 135–136
 see also individual policies
unpaid carers
 carer identity 2–3, 76–79, 116, 137
 carers assessments 79–83, 94, 138–139, 140, 141
 employment 4, 22, 33, 43, 44, 46, 48–49, 98, 124
 impact of caring on 2, 33
 lack of support for 8, 9, 10
 likelihood of becoming 115
 local planning and 70–73
 numbers of 76
  2001 Census 23
  Carers UK 15–16, 18, 24
  Family Resources Survey 2021 15
  General Household Surveys (GHS) 21, 22
  Scottish Census 24
  Social Market Foundation 24
 perception of 73–76, 107
 precarity 119–120, 126–127
 recognition of 120–121, 136–140
 relationships with professionals 89–91, 99
 rights agenda 48–51, 109–112, 136–140
 use of terminology 13, 14
 see also unpaid care: care relationships

V

Valuing Carers: A Strategy for Carers in Northern Ireland (DHSSPS 2002) 44, 47–48
voluntary sector 47, 71–73, 105, 106, 136
vulnerability 29, 31, 119, 127

W

Waerness, K. 121
Wales 10
 austerity policies 99–100
 Carer's Allowance 59
 carers assessments 80, 82, 140
 carers' involvement 70, 71
 devolution 40, 41, 97
 modernisation agenda 96
 numbers of unpaid carers 24
 personalisation agenda 51
 policies to support carers **37–38**, 43–44, 45–46, 47, 53–54, 54–56, 61–62, 78
 services and support for carers 67–68
Walker, A. 5, 10
Watson, N. 27
welfare funding 123
welfare reform 121
wellbeing 54
Wicks, M. 36
Wiles, J. 31
Williams, C. 96
Williams, F. 94–95
Willis, P.B. 72, 84
With Respect to Old Age: Long Term Care: Rights and Responsibilities (Royal Commission on Long Term Care, 1999) 75
women
 as carers 4, 5, 17, 18, 21, 22, 23, 124
 impact of austerity on 98
Wood, R. 6
Woolham, J. 89
Work and Families Act, 2006 58, 110

Y

Yeandle, S. 91, 94, 95
Young, H. 23

Z

Zhang, Y. 115

www.ingramcontent.com/pod-product-compliance
Lightning Source LLC
Chambersburg PA
CBHW071708020426
42333CB00017B/2189